Communication in the dental office

A PROGRAMMED MANUAL FOR THE DENTAL PROFESSIONAL

Communication in the dental office

A PROGRAMMED MANUAL FOR THE DENTAL PROFESSIONAL

ROBERT E. FROELICH, M.D., F.A.P.A.

Professor and Chairman of Psychiatry, Assistant Dean for
Program Development and Evaluation, School of Primary
Medical Care, The University of Alabama in Huntsville,
Huntsville, Alabama

F. MARIAN BISHOP, Ph.D., M.S.P.H.

Professor and Chairman of Community Medicine, School of Primary
Medical Care, The University of Alabama in Huntsville,
Huntsville, Alabama

SAMUEL F. DWORKIN, D.D.S., Ph.D.

Associate Dean for Academic Affairs, Professor of Oral Surgery
and Adjunct Professor of Psychiatry, University of Washington
School of Dentistry and School of Medicine, Seattle, Washington

Introduction by
Robert G. Hansen, D.D.S., M.P.H.
Dean and Professor, School of Dentistry,
Oral Roberts University, Tulsa, Oklahoma

The C. V. Mosby Company

Saint Louis   1976

GW/M/M 9 8 7 6 5 4

Preface

When a number of friends and acquaintances learned that *Communication in the Dental Office* was underway, most of their spontaneous responses were something like: "You're kidding!" "When did they get interested in that?" "But they are just mouth mechanics; they don't communicate." "Can I get a copy for my dentist?" "It's about time." The message seems to be that the consumer of dental services believes that communication in the dental office can be improved. We agree.

A recent experience exemplifies the problem. A dental surgeon extracted four wisdom teeth from a teenage patient. He called the mother in and said, "Everything is fine, and my assistant will tell you what to do." With that, he disappeared. The assistant gave the patient and his mother a rapid-fire series of instructions about what should be done to care for the patient and his mouth following the extractions. When they got in the car to go home, the mother asked, "Did you understand what she told you to do?"

"No, I didn't feel so hot, and I thought you were understanding what she was telling us," her son answered.

"Well, I didn't understand what she was saying either," the mother replied. "Her instructions didn't make sense, and she never stopped for questions."

The sad part of the story is that the dental assistant never knew what was heard by the patient and his mother. The assistant never took the extra 30 seconds to learn if they heard and how they interpreted what she said, or if they had any questions. And the dentist abdicated all responsibility of communication with the patient and his mother.

An audiotape recording of the assistant's instructions would probably be beyond criticism if written down. However, sending out words is only a small part of communication. This book is about communication, and it is about much more than just the sending out of words.

We want to give special thanks to Edwin F. Froelich, D.D.S., and John S. Rathbone, D.D.S., for their courage and willingness to share audiotape recordings made in their offices. These tapes were most valuable in the development of the sample interviews in this manual.

Robert E. Froelich

F. Marian Bishop

Samuel F. Dworkin

v

Contents

The need for effective communication in dentistry

ROBERT G. HANSEN, D.D.S.

Dentistry requires an exceptionally close physical proximity of two or more people. There is an obvious need for the dentist and the dental staff to maintain hand-to–face-and-mouth contact with the patient, and the treatment situation forces all of them into prolonged periods of being face to face and eye to eye. Adding intensity to the situation is the fact that all patients, to varying degrees, have anxieties about dental care. The dental chair places them in a position that is restraining and subordinate to that of the dental staff, and for some patients the oral cavity is an emotionally charged body area. Dentistry then, in an interpersonal sense, consists of a variety of people working together to provide intensely personal services to other people who are experiencing stress.

Even though most of dentistry involves interaction between people, these interactions receive relatively little study and attention in the profession. Unfortunately, the literature in dentistry deals almost entirely with dental diseases, methods and procedures of treatment, and delivery systems. Very little of a scientific nature has been written about the interpersonal factors of dentistry. Cohen and Richards, have observed that:

> Much of what passes for social science consists of arm-chair philosophy and of statements of subjective and personal beliefs which owe very little to scientific or objective method—this has been particularly so in the field of the dentist-patient relationship and communication. . . . There has been a plethora of anecdotal reminiscences on the part of individual practitioners on how to make the patient feel at ease, but very little empirical research to test out theory.*

Kruper reported in 1970 that at least 4 hours of communication skills were taught in about half of the schools responding to a questionnaire regarding teaching of behavioral sciences in schools of dentistry.† Since the reported mode

---

*Richards, D. N., and Cohen, L. K., editors: Social sciences and dentistry: a critical bibliography, © Federation Dentaire Internationale, The Hague, Netherlands, 1971, A. Sitjhoff International Publishing Co.
†Kruper, D. A.: Report on a behavioral science questionnaire sent to dental schools, presented to the Section on Community and Preventive Dentistry of the American Association of Dental Schools, New York, March 1970.

1

was 0 hours and the calculated mean was 7 hours, it is apparent that little formal attention has been devoted to developing student's abilities in this area. He noted that the data from the survey suggest that less than 1% of a student's time is spent on behavioral or social science. This situation occurs in spite of the recognition of the amount of time spent by a dentist in actual face-to-face contact with patients.

Since Kruper's report in 1970, interest in the behavioral sciences has increased. This increased interest has been greatly influenced by a promotion of preventive dentistry by the dental profession. Long espoused by the profession, preventive dentistry has taken on new importance and meaning; there has been an increased emphasis on the importance of removing plaque and on the necessity for motivating, educating, and training patients in effective personal oral cleaning practices. It has been recognized that for most persons to succeed in maintaining their natural dentition in good health and function throughout life, they must each day effectively remove virtually all of the dental plaque from their teeth with a toothbrush and dental floss. This placing of responsibility for oral health on each person has made it essential that the dentist and his staff become proficient in the difficult tasks of guiding patients in the performance of the required cleansing activities. The motivational and educational efforts involved in assisting patients to establish, and sometimes change, habit patterns and personal performances demand a high degree of insight and skill in communications. In response to this need there has been a greater emphasis in recent years on teaching communication skills to dental students, on establishing new societies concerned with preventive dentistry, on developing behavioral science sections in dental research and education associations, and on creating new journals and newsletters dealing with preventive dentistry and human behavior. There has also been a dramatic increase in presentations by behavioral scientists to dental groups on how to understand and communicate with patients.

After reviewing over 100 references concerning professional interest and practices in motivating patients toward sustained effective oral hygiene practices, Dr. Jeremy Shulman has concluded:

> Though there is no standardized procedure for long term oral hygiene motivation, present knowledge does suggest that the approach which should be used today would be first, the establishment of communication; second, an attempt to evaluate each patient in terms of possible motivational incentives; third, the use of a variety of motivational techniques based on the empirical assessment of each patient's needs; fourth, repetition of the instruction; fifth, varied reinforcements of desired behavior, and lastly, the use of those mechanical aids which have been shown to have potential value.*

A common thread in the dental literature on human behavior and interpersonal relations is that effective communication, whether it is for effective and efficient staff function or for enhancing the doctor-patient relation and providing the best possible care for the patient, is essential to success in the dental office.

Communication and rapport, essential for understanding and trust, form the very essence of the doctor-patient relationship. However, humor frequently depicts the dentist as carrying on a one-way conversation (including questions)

---

*Shulman, J.: Current concepts of patient motivation toward long term oral hygiene: a literature review, J. Am. Soc. Prev. Dent. 4(6):7-15, 1974.

with a patient whose mouth is filled with paraphernalia preventing a reply. The message is clear: dentists are not viewed as persons excelling in meaningful communication.

The dental office as a therapeutic setting for oral health presents an inherent danger of focusing attention on a limited physical part of the individual rather than on the whole person. Although a dentist's special professional abilities are in the realm of dental health, to concentrate only on the dental condition would be to ignore personal and behavioral factors that contribute to the current dental status and most certainly have a role in determining future conditions and behavior.

Communication actually begins or at least is conditioned before any verbal exchange between a dentist and a patient takes place. The circumstances of the patient seeking professional attention and selecting a specific practitioner involve a host of factors that lead to certain anxieties and expectations and create a unique psychologic stance when verbal communication begins.

Success in a dental practice depends in large measure on the quality of the dentist-patient relationship. When expressing reasons for utilizing a certain dentist, patients mention the personal qualities of a dentist just as frequently as they do his technical excellence. It is probable that in most cases a patient goes to a dentist who the patient likes; the patient then attributes technical competence to the dentist, since it is virtually impossible for a patient to really know the quality of technical services rendered by the dentist. Moreover, much of the time the patient cannot actually see the results of the dentist's work.

Teeth and the oral cavity have a profound effect on a person's entire life. Dworkin has said:

> Extensive decay, tooth loss or malfunction may have led to behavioral patterns of withdrawal, embarrassment, interference with normal speech patterns, change in eating habits, etc. . . . Contemplating dental treatment may arouse castration anxiety, aging neurosis, or orally related anxieties.*

Through sucking and eating the oral cavity is the locus of the first human experiences of pleasure and satisfaction, and through teething it is one of the first areas of pain.

The oral cavity is the most concentrated area of sensation in infancy; besides the pain and the pleasure it offers, the oral cavity is used for investigation and sensation through touch and taste, as well as for verbal and nonverbal expression. The extent of the continuation of the oral phase into adult life and implications for the care of patients in the oral area have not been fully investigated by behavioral scientists, but it is obvious that the psychologic implications of the oral phase for dental care and the doctor-patient relationship can be significant.

In dental periodicals numerous authors describe the importance of, and the ways to identify, personality types and psychologic characteristics of patients. The influences of fear, anxiety, and aspects of orality on patient behavior are repeatedly noted. Frequently, advice is offered on how to manage various kinds of patients and on how to use various psychologic techniques and existential orientations to relate to and motivate patients. Some solutions to the problems of communication and for improving the doctor-patient relationship appear

---

*Dworkin, S. F.: Psychomatic concepts and dentistry: some perspectives, J. Periodontol. **40:**647-654, 1967.

overly simplistic, and others suggest a complexity requiring the dental professional to be a chameleon, responding to every patient in a unique way appropriate for that patient. An experienced clinical psychologist would be hard pressed to even come close to achieving the insight and expertise in therapeutic interpersonal relations that some authors promote for the dental professional. It is essential, however, for optimal care of the patient and professional satisfaction of the dentist and dental staff, that effective communication be established. The procedures and methods in this book are designed to provide practical and useful techniques for achieving the level of communications necessary to achieve therapeutic and preventive results and satisfying dentist-patient-staff relationships.

Although socioeconomic classes differ in their attitudes, beliefs, and practices concerning dental health, most people believe that heredity, luck, and diet have more effect on dental health than dental care or their own hygiene practices.* This situation is beginning to change, however, and in the last 10 years an enthusiasm has developed within the dental profession for preventive dentistry, which places a strong emphasis on making patients responsible for their own dental health. Therefore, dental professionals must assume an added function, that of being effective educators, motivators, and trainers of patients in proper oral health practices. Many dental professionals become discouraged and frustrated when they experience minimal success in significantly altering the oral hygiene practices of their patients.†

There is a marked contrast between the way most of the public view dental health and the way dental professionals view dental health. Although both groups consider teeth important, the degree of importance is vastly different; the public generally has a fatalistic attitude that teeth will eventually cause trouble and pain and will have to be removed. The inevitability of tooth loss is not shared by dentists who practice a modern concept of preventive dentistry and maintenance of the dentition. The dental professional views good dental health as important because of the relationship of dental health with general and emotional health and because of the importance of a sound dentition for mastication, speech, comfort, and appearance. The public rarely is consciously aware of the importance of good dental health in relation to these factors and incorrectly concludes that loosing teeth is not very important because of a mistaken belief that replacing natural teeth with dentures yields good results.

Dental services are obtained annually by less than 50% of the population of the United States, and much of this care is limited in scope or is urgent intervention to relieve pain or infection, or both. Probably no more than 20% of the people receive regular or comprehensive care to maintain optimal oral health. Dental professionals believe that the dentition of virtually everyone can be maintained in good health and function throughout life by a combination of fluoridation of water, good personal oral hygiene practices, and regular preventive and therapeutic care by a dentist. However, well over 20 million people age 18 to 79 are completely endentulous, and the most recent national study, conducted in 1960

---

*Bureau of Economic Research and Statistics: A motivation study of dental care, J. Am. Dent. Assoc. **56:**434-443, 566-574, 745-751, 911-917, 1958.
†Press release, Bureau of Public Information, American Dental Association, March 25, 1974.

to 1962, revealed that the rest of the population had an average of 18 decayed, filled, and missing teeth.* The missing teeth had been removed because long-neglected decay and other diseases had destroyed the teeth or the health of the supporting tissues. There is no reason to believe that the overall situation is any better in 1975, although the preventive benefits of fluoridation are being noted in younger age groups. Effective as fluoridation is, however, it does not prevent all dental caries and only has an indirect effect on other dental diseases and conditions.

Morris has noted that it is essential for the dental professional to have an accurate understanding and assessment of latent demands for dental care as well as of the customarily described absolutes of need and demand. He believes that with education, legislation, and social planning, the argument concerning the discrepancy between needs and active demands would become moot. Morris has decribed a spectrum of patients by a descending order of dental awareness as follows:

1. Patients who demand and receive dental care.
2. Patients who demand (make an effort to obtain) dental care but, for various reasons, are unable to obtain it.
3. Patients (or their parents) who recognize the need and articulate the desire for dental care but do not, in fact, actively seek it.
4. Patients who personally acknowledge existence of dental disease and consciously recognize need for treatment but do not articulate need.
5. Patients who are conscious that dental disease exists but do not recognize that treatment is indicated.
6. Patients who are unaware of existing dental diseases.
7. Patients without dental disease who do not recognize the need for preventive services or procedures.†

Since relatively few people are in the first category, it is apparent that most people do not consider dental services essential and that few consider dental disease serious. In fact, many view the obtaining of dental services as an unpleasant and costly inconvenience that they frequently deeply resent. Such persons may also view the dentist as a sadistic, greedy mechanic who works on teeth. The implications of such views on dentist-patient communication are obviously profound.

The first visit to a dental office sets the stage for all future visits, since a patient forms attitudes in anticipation of and during the first visit. Rapport must be established as soon as possible. Delay in establishing rapport can make future constructive exchange more difficult. Auxiliary personnel in the dental office contribute significantly to the tone and level of communication that is established.

One crucial function of communication in the dental office is to secure information concerning the patient and the patient's dental condition. In 1974 Kegeles, speaking on preventive care practices, to the Sixty-second Annual World

---

*National Center for Health Statistics: Selected dental findings in adults by age, race, and sex, United States 1960-1962 Vital and Health Statistics, PHS Publ. 1,000–Series II, No. 7, Public Health Service, Washington, D.C., 1965, Government Printing Office.
†Morris, A. L.: Training and utilization of dental manpower. In Brown, W. E., editor: Oral health, dentistry and the American public: the need for an improved oral care delivery system, Norman, Okla., 1974, University of Oklahoma Press.

Congress of the Federation Dentaire International, suggested that eight pieces of information should be obtained from patients. They are:

> (1) The previous frequency of visits and the reasons for the visits by the patient because "the best single predictor of dental behavior is past dental behavior"; (2) the patient's knowledge about relationships between tooth brushing, dental visits, home care, and dental caries or periodontal disease so he can be educated in the gaps in his knowledge; (3) his previous experience with dentists so that the dentist will not repeat actions that have made the patient unhappy in the past; (4) the economic, educational, and occupational status of the patient so that the dentist will know what the patient can afford to pay for his care; (5) the previous preventive medical care undertaken by the patient, because preventive behavior is similar in medical and dental areas; (6) the dental behavior of the patient's family, which tends to be similar to his; (7) the attitudes of patients toward the importance of dentistry and their chances of having serious dental problems, including loss of teeth; (8) the extent of tolerance of pain and anxiety about treatment to determine the amount of reassurance the patient may need and the type of anesthetic to be used.*

Although the items are not comprehensive for all dental conditions and problems, such information is essential for the dentist to know enough about the patient to be able to effectively plan and implement treatment. In addition to gaining information to help plan treatment, an extensive medical-dental-social history assists the dental professional in understanding factors that motivate patients to seek care and factors that possibly interfere with patients carrying out home care. The diagnostic information obtained through communication is as important to diagnosis and treatment planning as is the information obtained through the physical examination of the oral cavity. In addition, the action of a patient communicating the details of his/her dental history and experience functions to help allay fears, tensions, and anxieties.

Because all individuals are continuously susceptible to dental diseases, most people will experience a continuous, periodic need for treatment from the time the teeth erupt in the mouth. Three unique characteristics of the two most common diseases of the mouth (dental caries and periodontal disease), accounting for some of the structure and organization of the dental profession, are:

1. They are of almost universal prevalence.
2. They do not undergo remission or termination if untreated but accumulate a backlog of unmet needs.
3. They almost always require technically demanding, expensive and time-consuming surgical and prosthetic professional treatment and rarely will respond to professional advice, prescription, or medication.†

These unique features have contributed to the development of a dental profession separate from, rather than a conventional speciality within, the practice of medicine. The dental profession in the United States could be considered to have originated during the years 1839 and 1840, since it was during these years that the first dental school was founded, the first dental periodical in the world began publication, and the first national group of dentists was formed.‡ By

---

*FDI session explores optimum operation of dental team, Oct. 7, 1974, ADA News, p. 6.
†Young, W. O.: Dentistry looks toward the twenty-first century. In Brown, W. E., editor: Oral health, dentistry and the American public: the need for an improved oral care delivery system, Norman, Okla., 1974. University of Oklahoma Press.
‡Bremmer, M. D. K.: The story of dentistry. In Dawn of civilization to the present, ed. 2, Brooklyn, 1946, Dental Items of Interest.

1868 several states had passed laws governing the practice of dentistry. From the beginning the profession had autonomy through control of its educational institutions, scientific literature, and professional organizations, and through separate licensing authority.

Some dentists who had been trained through apprenticeships to established practitioners opposed the first schools for the training of dentists, whereas others saw the potential for profit as preceptors and established proprietary schools. The proprietary schools flourished for several decades, largely replacing apprenticeship training, until the 1926 report on dental education conducted by William Gies. This report reinforced the efforts of the American Dental Association to upgrade the standards of education. Thereafter, many proprietary schools closed. Others, however, became affiliated with universities. Now, all dental schools are affiliated with universities and are accredited by the Council on Dental Education of the American Dental Association, and all graduates must satisfy the requirements of a state-licensing board before being permitted to practice. The licensing boards have traditionally been composed of members of the dental profession, although some consumer and legal challenges to this practice are developing.

During the first half of the 1970s, a number of monographs and journal articles have appeared, reporting studies and observations on the past, present, and future of dentistry. Prominent among these have been collections of articles written on several themes by a number of distinguished authors. They include *Oral Health, Dentistry and the American Public*, edited by W. E. Brown; *Toward a Sociology of Dentistry*, edited by R. M. O'Shea and L. K. Cohen; *Group Practice and the Future of Dental Care*, edited by C. R. Jerge, W. E. Marshall, M. H. Schoen, and J. W. Frieman; and *Social Sciences and Dentistry: A Critical Bibliography*, by N. D. Richards and L. K. Cohen.* These publications contain extensive reviews and summaries of the literature, which together give a comprehensive description of the dynamics of dental practice in the 1970s in the United States. To give some perspective to the setting of dental office communication, this introduction briefly summarizes some of the information presented in these publications. A thorough reading of the publications would be instructive and rewarding to any dentist or student desiring more insight and understanding of the profession.

One of the most highly prized features of being a dentist is the opportunity to be one's own boss. The pattern of dentists practicing alone in their own offices without partners and with no sharing of costs has predominated; in 1973 nearly 65% of dentists practiced in that manner with an average of one to two dental auxiliaries per office.† Approximately 10% were self-employed without partners but shared some costs. Only 3% to 5% of dentists practiced in groups defined

---

*Brown, W. E., editor: Oral health, dentistry and the American public: the need for an improved oral care delivery system, Norman, Okla., 1974, University of Oklahoma Press; O'Shea, R. M., and Cohen, L. K. editors: Toward a sociology of dentistry, The Milbank Memorial Fund Quarterly 49(3):336, 1971; Jerge, C. R., Marshall, W. E., Schoen, M. H., and Friedman, J. W., editors: Group practice and the future of dental care, Philadelphia, 1974, Lea & Febiger; Richards, N. D., and Cohen, L. K., editors: Social sciences and dentistry: a critical bibliography, © Federation Dentaire Internationale, The Hague, Netherlands, 1971, A. Sijhoff International Publishing Co.
†Gies, W. J.: Dental education in the United States and Canada, New York, 1926, Carnegie Foundation for Advanced Teaching.

as "... a practice formally organized to provide care through the services of three or more dentists using office space, equipment and/or personnel jointly."[*] Group practice does show some signs of growing; this situation is perhaps influenced by the fact that establishing a dental practice is so costly, averaging more than $28,000 in 1973.[†]

The nature of dental practice requires the constant use of expensive, complex, and specialized technical equipment and the assistance of specially trained auxiliary personnel. These factors tend to keep dentistry from the forms of organization and closer affiliations found with medicine, because in medicine the more complex facilities, auxiliary personnel, and equipment are used more sporadically, can be shared, and are frequently provided by other entities in the community; the obvious example is the hospital with its sophisticated surgical, custodial, and medical technology facilities and extensive and diverse personnel.

Another important difference between medical and dental care is the method of financing the care. Young has analyzed a number of surveys and reports and has concluded that 90% of the cost of dental care is financed privately by individuals receiving the care and that less than 10% is covered by third party sources, including insurance and government.[‡] In a social security study it is reported that about 60% of total health service expenses for those persons under age 65 and about 75% of the expenses for those 65 and over are paid by third parties.[§] Since there is little optimism that dental services will be included in any enactment of a national health insurance program, the financing picture is not expected to change markedly in the immediate future; however, some funds now committed to various types of health and hospitalization insurance programs could possibly be redirected to dental prepayment programs if these services were to be included in a national health insurance act. The direct payment for most dental services tends to contribute toward the consideration of dentistry as an optional or nonessential health service.

The need of a dentist to secure information about patients and their dental experiences, conditions, and attitudes will continue, as will the needs to discuss proposed treatments and to reach agreements on charges and the details of payment, to educate, motivate, and train patients in attitudes and performances concerning effective oral hygiene practices, to perform necessary treatment, to collaborate with other dentists and health practitioners, to supervise and sometimes train auxiliary personnel, to manage a small business, and to be a professional who is a citizen in the community. Dentistry is a complex profession with many demands and responsibilities but also with many rewards and satisfactions. Personal enjoyment and the provision of the best possible services for patients depend on many factors; since so much of dental practice involves interactions between the dentist, the patients, and the staff, however, communication skills are essential for success.

[*]Bureau of Economic Research and Statistics: American Dental Association 1971 Survey of dental practices: II. Income of dentists by location, age and other factors, J. Am. Dent. Assoc. **84:**397-402, 1972.
[†]U.S. Public Health Service: Dental group practice in the United States, 1971, a survey, Washington, D.C., 1972, Department of Health, Education, and Welfare.
[‡]Bureau of Economic Research and Statistics: American Dental Association survey of recent dental graduates, J. Am. Dent. Assoc. **87:**1248-1250, 1973.
[§]Cooper, B. S., and Worthington, N.: Medical care spending for three age groups, Social security Bulletin **35:**3-16, 1972.

SECTION I COMMUNICATION PRELIMINARIES

1 Choosing the dental office

Most problems dentists and staff have with patients are not related to the physical, biologic, and technical aspects of dental practices. It is the human aspect of the dentist, the dental staff, and the patient that interferes with the utilization of dental knowledge and skills. The dentist, the dental staff, and the patient are all products of their various social-cultural backgrounds and their own unique life experiences. As a result, they have different norms, values, and expectations about life in general and about the dental interaction in particular. These differences, if unrecognized, can lead to misunderstandings and complications between the dentist, the dental staff, and the patient. We believe that when dental professionals are alert to differing expectations, they are in a better position to divert potential problems and complications. The needs, assumptions, and expectations imposed on the patient by the dentist, the dental staff, and the physical environment will also influence how and when the communication process begins and how well it proceeds. This situation is especially true during the first appointment.

Sensitivity to, and understanding of, the patient's entering behavior, along with the dentist's awareness of his/her own biases and expectations, will reduce conflict and anxiety and will facilitate the establishment of individualized ground rules for the dentist-patient interaction. With less conflict and anxiety and mutually accepted ground rules, relevant diagnostic information can be elicited in a more efficient manner. A major concern of dentists is that patients are satisfied and will return. This concern influences how the dentist and dental staff listen and talk to patients.

Question: Within the context of dental communications, what is meant by the *entering behavior* of the patient?

Answer: The patient's entering behavior provides clues as to why the patient has come and are indications of the patient's anxiety level, expectations, background, and willingness to accept mutually agreeable ground rules. We deal with the details of these nonverbal clues in Section III.

Question: How does obtaining such knowledge fit in with the general purpose of a dental interview?

Answer: The purpose of the dental interview can be summarized as a strategy for allowing you, the dental professional, with your own needs and expectancies, to identify the needs of your patients and the conflicts your patients may have over having those needs met. The end result is to be able to plan and execute effective and efficient behaviors, on the part of both yourself and the patient, that allow needs to be met under positively reinforcing conditions.

Question: In any given year about how many Americans visit a dentist at least once?

Answer: About 40% of Americans see a dentist at least once a year. However, the proportion of people under regular dental care is much lower. In any event, one clear obstacle to communication is the fact that the majority of Americans do not go to the dentist regularly.

Question: Using the format below, list the factors that may be a source of conflict and that contribute to the patient's decision to go or not to go to the dentist. Under each factor give examples of reasons patients may give for going or not going.

To go	Not to go

Answer: The following reasons may be given by a patient for going or not going to the dentist.

To go	Not to go

A. *Previous personal dental history*

To go	Not to go
A positive experience. Liked the dentist. Didn't experience any discomfort during treatment. Needs met with individual attention. Questions answered. Fees reasonable and adequately explained.	Traumatic experience. Really hurt. Little or no explanation. No personal attention. Cost too much. Too much talk and too little work. Questions not answered.

B. *Cultural, ethnic, socioeconomic factors*

To go	Not to go
White, middle-class Americans expected to go to dentist regularly. Teeth an important part of appearance in this society. Important to take care of my body. Bad teeth can poison the rest of my system. Money spent on maintaining good oral health is well worth it.	Teeth aren't important, anyhow. I could have them all out and have a plate made. Doctors and dentists rip off people. Going to the dentist is a waste of money; it's really not so important.

C. Psychosocial factors

Pain perception

I'll feel better if I go now, when nothing is hurting me.

Pain is so difficult for me to endure, I'll do anything to avoid it.

Uncertainty

He probably won't tell me anything I don't know.

I can't stand not knowing what's going to happen next. When the dentist is working on me, I think, "It doesn't hurt now, but maybe it soon will."

Perceived illness

If the dentist finds out there's something wrong, it's good that I know and start corrective procedures.

If something's wrong, I don't want to know. I get very anxious over the possibility that a part of my body isn't functioning properly or isn't in good health.

Body image

My body's an important concern. I'm very interested in keeping my body in good shape.

I don't like the idea of anyone tampering with my body or even touching me physically unless I know that person very well.

Authority

Dentists and doctors are good because they take charge and take care of me.

Who needs them? Dentists and doctors seem to have a need to control people. I don't see why I should give in to them unless I have to.

You may have listed additional sources of conflict for a person contemplating going to a dentist. Reviewing these conflicts should increase your awareness of potential concerns that a patient may have.

Question: Are all sources of potential conflict equally observable?

Answer: No. Some of these sources are readily elicited by simple questions and observations. Other sources of conflict, especially the psychosocial ones, may not be readily observable and may have to be interpreted from the patient's responses. We are constantly interpreting or inferring attitudes and feelings from what people say. However, to ensure that your interpretations are correct and that you are not being led astray by your own conflicts or needs, it is best to check your interpretations or inferences with the patient.

Mr. Arthur comes to your dental office after selecting your name out of a telephone book because of the convenient location. Mr. Baker comes to your office on the basis of a recommendation from a personal friend. He has been told something about how your office is run, what kind of person you are, what to expect on the first visit, and even what you billed the friend for fees.

Question: Why is this information important to you, the dentist?

Answer: The specific factors that help a person resolve conflicts into a decision to see a particular dentist affect the understanding between the dentist and the patient and are very important in determining how the two people approach each other.

Question: Why might a patient select a particular dentist?

Answer: A patient might select a particular dentist for the following reasons:
1. The office is located in a geographically convenient or prestigious area.
2. The dentist has a reputation for excellent clinical dentistry— the things the dentist does have good results.
3. The patient thinks the dentist is thorough in examination and maintenance of oral health.
4. The patient perceives the dentist as being approachable, a "nice person," easy to talk to (and may give little thought or concern to the level or quality of dentistry that the dentist is supposed to be able to perform).
5. The dentist is reputed to be *concerned* with the overall health of the patient, is available for complete explanations, and is willing to answer questions concerning the progress of the work and difficulties that may arise.

It appears that some people assume and expect to be satisfied patients primarily through good clinical dentistry. Other patients assume and expect the source of their satisfaction to be primarily through the development of a relationship with a dental health authority figure. Although this categorization is somewhat oversimplified, it reflects the way many people speak about their dentists; therefore, it reflects the needs they have when they go for treatment.

Question: Is it only the patient who has needs and assumptions, and expectancies? Does the dentist have a similar set of needs, assumptions, and expectancies that determine how he/she will begin and and maintain a communication process with patients?

Answer: Definitely. If the dentist is competent clinically, then whether his/her needs, assumptions, and expectancies (of having a successful dental practice) are met depend on the dentist's ability to elicit cooperative patient behavior and develop satisfying long-term relationships. The cooperative patient is generally thought of as being able to understand and accept the need for specified treatment procedures, is psychologically or pharmacologically capable of tolerating clinical procedures, and is reasonably reliable. Although the need for long-term relationships vary according to the specialty areas of practice (for example, long-term relationships with patients may not be a major concern of the oral surgeon, who frequently sees patients only once or twice), a predominant expectancy of the general dentist is that in most cases an enduring dentist-patient relationship can be developed that will persist over time.

2 Initial contact with the dental office

The patient has decided to contact a dental office for care. Consider, for a moment, the patient's state of mind.

Question: How would you describe the patient's state of mind? (How do you feel when you are about to embark on a new experience in a new territory?)

Answer: The most universal reaction to a new situation or new people at a time when you are asking for help, feeling a little helpless, and needing to depend on someone else whom you don't yet know is anxiety. The degree of anxiety depends on a number of variables: How many different experiences with new people have you encountered before? (Did you grow up in a community where you knew everyone and rarely met a stranger?) How secure are you within yourself? Are you really okay? Can you really handle any situation? What thoughts do you have about a new situation that might scare you?

Some patient's feel trapped and intruded on because they have to break their routine and go to a dental office. They don't like the intrusion into their life. They are annoyed and frustrated because the appointment prevents them from continuing toward their planned goal. They may be angered. They don't like being sick, having pain, or not being perfect. Thus, the receptionist may be confronted with anger, unexplained aggression, irritability, or a contrary patient.

Still other patients will view their need for dental care as a loss of their integrity, a loss of their wholeness, a loss of their power, and possibly a loss of their youth. For some, losing teeth is the first sign of getting old. These patients will react with some degree of grief and sadness. Their spirits will be down, and there may be some slowing of their normal physiologic functioning. Extreme slowing of physiologic functioning leads to coating of the tongue, constipation, decreased salivation, dryness of mouth, and slowed movements, such as in gait, gestures, and speech. This extreme slowing will not occur from just the need for a dental appointment, but if the dental appointment is part of other losses, such as losses from a death, business, divorce, or the like, the changes in the general physiology may lead to changes in the environment of the mouth to the point that changes begin to occur in the gums, bone, and teeth. Examples of these changes can be found in state mental hospitals in people who have had long periods of altered physiologic responses.

Question: With the patient in a state of mind somewhere within the range of feelings just reviewed, what is the job of the dental office receptionist when the phone rings?

Answer: The receptionist's job is to establish communication with the prospective patient in such a way that the appointment will be made and kept.

Question: Assume that the patient is experiencing some anxiety and has some of the other feelings. What does the prospective patient want to hear on the telephone?

Answer: The patient wants the telephone voice on the other end to be concerned, accepting of them and their feelings, and warm and friendly rather than cold, distant, and businesslike.

Question: Listed below are ways to answer an office telephone. Select the one(s) you prefer.
A. 345-4673.
B. Doctor's office.
C. Hello.
D. Dr. Howard West's office, Kathy speaking.
E. Dr. Howard West's office, Kathy Arnold speaking.
F. Dr. West's office, Ms. Arnold speaking.
G. Dr. West's.
H. Dr. West's office, may I help you?

Answer: We prefer *D, E,* and *F.*
A is cold and distant.
B doesn't inform you whether you have reached the correct doctor's office.
C could very easily be inferred as "Hello, stop bothering me."
G is a step in the right direction but continues to be impersonal.
H is friendly, gives information, and is acceptable.

We prefer for the receptionist to give her name. When the receptionist gives her name, the caller usually does likewise without having to be asked for it. When we give our names, we are saying that we are individuals, that we are not ashamed of our names, that we stand behind our names, and by inference, that we stand behind what we do. Giving our name makes our conversations personal rather than impersonal. It also implies that we deal with unique individuals who have names, not with abstract, depersonalized patients.

The next job of the receptionist is to obtain the caller's name and request. The receptionist needs to record the request as accurately as possible, because what the caller says contains clues as to the caller's state of mind, what he/she really wants (not just what he/she wants on the surface), and what concerns he/she has.

Question: How should the receptionist ask the patient for the reason for the appointment?
A. Why do you want the appointment?
B. What trouble do you have?
C. What is bothering you?
D. What may I record as your reason for the appointment?
E. May I indicate on your record your reason for the appointment?

Answer: *D* and *E* are the preferred answers. These questions infer that the receptionist will listen to what is said in reply, is concerned with what is about to be said, and will write down what is said. They suggest that no judgment will be made regarding the legitimacy of the patient's request for an appointment.
A tends to be accusative and places the patient in a defensive position to justify the request for an appointment.
B and *C* are too superficial for a professional setting.

Question: Consider each of the following responses to the receptionist's question, "What may I record as your reason for the appointment?" Which patient is anxious? Which patient is angry? Which patient is sad?
A. I (pause) I have a toothache. (Said at the beginning of expiration.)
B. I need an appointment for my toothache. (Said forcefully.)
C. My tooth hurts. (Said slowly at the end of expiration.)

Answer: *A* is anxious.
B is angry.
C is sad.

Note that the pause and how the voice sounds are part of the communication and need to be recorded by the receptionist. The hesitations, voice quality, respiration, and so on, may be more important than what the patient says, in terms of how soon you see the patient, how you deal with the patient, and what treatment you recommend. If the patient is so angry that his/her teeth are constantly under the pressure of a tight masseter muscle, your planned treatment may have to be altered. Similarly, if there isn't sufficient salivary flow to keep an acrylic filling moistened, your treatment will also need to be changed. But more important, you might not want to make jokes with the angry patient or expect the sad patient to actively pursue dental exercises. You know that the anxious, somewhat hysterical patient, on the other hand, will overdo your suggestions in his/her attempt to please you.

The receptionist should get the information from the patient that is available and make sure that the patient feels welcomed and cared for, so that the patient will keep the appointment and be in a state of mind that is conducive to good dental care.

There are differing opinions concerning the correct method and style to be used by the dental professional in meeting a new patient and in establishing an interview relationship of trust and confidence:

Should you personally escort the patient from the waiting room?

Should you have the patient wait in the operatory chair?

Should you first see the new patient in a private office setting?

Should you shake hands, or should you ignore this social convention?

Should you talk about the weather, or should you get right to the dental problem?

There is no single answer to these questions, since no single practice is accepted by all dental offices.

In the next frames assume that you (a patient) have just moved to a new city.

After telephoning a dental office and being told to come right in, that the dentist will see you about your throbbing tooth, you enter the office. The receptionist takes your name, address, occupation, complaint, and other information. She hangs up your coat and places you in the operatory chair and leaves the room. You wait for 50 minutes, and the dentist enters.

Question: As a patient, what is your reaction to this introduction to the office?

Answer: This introduction may leave you feeling that the office has an efficient receptionist but wondering if anyone has any interest in you.

Remember, many patients consider evidence of interest in them as a criterion of scientific competence. Every cultural group considers it insulting to be kept waiting beyond a certain period of time without some additional communication from office personnel. With alertness, the dental staff can determine what this time limit is for the individual community where the practice is located.

After telephoning a dental office and being told to come right in, that the dentist will see you about your throbbing tooth, you enter his office. The receptionist obtains the necessary information and asks you to be seated in the waiting room. After approximately 10 minutes the receptionist checks with the dentist and tells you that the dentist will be delayed in seeing you. She asks if she can make you more comfortable while you wait. After another 15 minutes the dentist introduces himself to you at the waiting room door, escorts you to the operatory, and takes your coat.

Question: As a patient, what is your reaction to this introduction to the office?

Answer: This introduction shows interest and respect on the part of the dental office. You are kept informed about a delayed time schedule. You know the dental staff is aware of your existence and uncomfortable state.

Being met in the office waiting room may lead to an awkward walk to the operatory chair, however. You cannot tell the dentist about your throbbing tooth in the hall. Depending on the length of the hall, this walk may be either comfortable or awkward.

After telephoning a dental office to ask about help for your throbbing tooth, you are told that the dentist can see you at 4:45 PM, but that if you become too uncomfortable, you may come in earlier and wait until you can be worked into the schedule. You enter the office 5 minutes before your appointment time. The receptionist obtains the necessary information. She hangs up your coat and places you in an operatory chair. The dentist enters at 4:47 and introduces himself.

Question: As a patient, what is your reaction to this introduction to the office?

Answer: This introduction shows concern about the value of the patient's time and understanding that the patient must weigh the degree of discomfort against spending time waiting in the dental office. You may appreciate the promptness and businesslike approach of the dental staff. Whether the dentist is a cold, unfeeling technician or a warm, understanding person will be shown by how he proceeds from here.

Each office develops a pattern of dealing with patients. Sometimes this pattern evolves by chance and with little or no thought given to the impression it gives to the patient. The dental staff should be aware of the way the patient is managed, including during the initial telephone contact, when the patient arrives at the office and during the initial face-to-face meeting with the patient. First impressions are too important to be left to chance.

Discussions with other professionals about these three examples and others that you may think of will further your understanding of how the patient reacts to office introductions. Such discussions should improve your control of the introduction patterns developed in your office.

The roles of the dental staff and the patient are defined by cultural definitions and expectations. The relationship is defined as a professional-client one, with certain reciprocal rights and privileges denied social relationships. The relationship between the dental staff and the patient is not a social one. Some dentists feel strongly that, from the outset, the behavior of the dentist should clearly indicate that the relationship is a professional one. It has a purpose that is agreed to by both the patient and the dentist and rarely is some social exchange necessary to begin the diagnostic interview. If the patient is unusually anxious, apprehensive, or frightened, then an element of social amenity might not be remiss.

Question: When meeting a new patient in your office, should you shake hands?

Answer: Social handshaking occurs primarily when two men meet initially or when they have been apart for some time. Shaking hands is much less frequent among women, although it is presently increasing as a feminine behavior. Shaking hands in a dentist's office is not common. After all, it is not a sociable relationship. On the other hand, you may obtain some valuable information from the handshake (whether the patient's hand is limp or firm, wet or dry, steady or shaking, clumsy or agile, deformed or normal) and can transmit your reaction to the patient (concern, support, considerateness, firmness, tenderness, or distance). The rule is to *shake hands if it is the comfortable thing* for you and for the patient to do.

19

3 Office settings

ENVIRONMENT

As the patient enters a new environment, his/her impression is based on the total sensory experience—temperature, colors, texture, sounds, location, dress, and artifacts. Some dental offices have a formal setting, whereas others are informal. Either an efficient, long-life, strong, durable, hard-surfaced rug or a soft, fluffy, well-padded inviting rug may be placed on the waiting room floor. The magazines may be *Playboy, Better Homes and Gardens, Popular Mechanics, Field and Stream, Children's Highlights,* or *National Geographic,* depending on your clientele. An inappropriate magazine for the social ethnic class may attract or repel patients as much as your technical skills.

Do you want to have games in the waiting room? Should you always have a half-finished puzzle on the table? What do you want the patient to do while waiting for you? Do you want to distract his/her thoughts? The waiting room may be a significant factor concerning how the patient will first respond to you.

Question: What do you want to say with your waiting room?
    A. This is a place of business; we are all business.
    B. We are friendly, and we are concerned with your comfort.
    C. You are welcome. Come in and be yourself.
    D. Come in. We don't trust you, so we have indestructable furniture.
    E. Come in and relax. Enjoy yourself while you wait.
    F. Be yourself; you are okay just the way you are.

Answer: We believe that you have the opportunity to say whatever you wish with the decor of the room and the artifacts placed there. Many people will read the message unconsciously, and a few will read it consciously. Either way, they will react to it and set the stage for their contact with you. The communication of the waiting room should be consistent with the style of the staff and the dentist. An "all business" waiting room should go with an "all business" staff and dentist.

Communication is affected by the relative positions of the persons communicating. The transactional positions of "I count" or "I don't count" is important for each person and can be manipulated by furniture. When one person, like

20

the judge in a courtroom, is seated above the other(s), the setting is a dominant-submissive ("I count—you don't count," or "parent-child") one. The position of the dental stool in relation to the dental chair may have a profound effect on some patients.

Question: What position, relative to yourself, do you want to encourage in the patient?
A. An equal position
B. A superior, dominant position
C. An inferior position

Answer: What fits your style? What will help get the current job done? Although the initial position affects the patient, it is not permanent. You can change this position as the type of treatment changes. As a rule the patient comes to a professional in a dependent position. Hopefully, as time progresses, the patient will grow and become more independent, more responsible for his own dental care and hygiene. The answer to this question then becomes one of what do you want to encourage at each stage of treatment? Once you decide, manipulate the setting to encourage that behavior on the part of the patient.

Generally, unless the difference in eye level of two people is more than 6 inches, the two people need to be in physically equivalent positions to allow for communication on an equal level and to encourage a mutual sharing of responsibility. This situation is in marked contrast to that of the patient lying flat on his/her back with the dental professional bending over the patient.

Question: What position do you want the patient to be in when you tell him/her what you want him/her to do to take care of the current dental treatment?

Answer: You want the patient in an upright position with feet firmly planted on the floor. The patient is then in a position to accept responsibility and respond to what he/she is told.*

PERSONNEL

Dentists recognize that the most efficient and effective dental care is given to patients when *auxiliary personnel,* such as receptionists, dental assistants, and dental hygienists, are employed. As the dentist is able to increasingly delegate functions that he/she used to do, his/her role changes to increasingly emphasize diagnosis, treatment planning, and the direct treatment services that only the dentist may perform.

Not all dental offices employ the same number and type of dental auxiliaries, but if even just one such person is employed, then there is created between the dentist, patient, and auxiliary a new and different set of relationships that directly affect communication in the dental treatment setting. Typically, the first person a patient communicates with when he/she approaches a particular treatment setting is *not* the dentist.

As more roles are filled by different people in the dental setting, the com-

---

*See Chapter 10 for elaboration of these ideas.

munication network becomes progressively complex. A desirable communication network for an office with only one dentist, a dental assistant, and a dental hygienist is shown below.

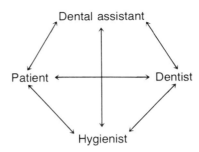

Entirely different kinds of psychologic and physical factors operate when a communication network extends to more than two people. Feelings of being left out, difficulty in maintaining eye contact, and errors in transmission of information (for example, concerning appointments or treatment to be rendered) increase dramatically as the number of people involved in the communication network is expanded.

The positive aspects of increased communication opportunities should not be overlooked. It is more likely that someone—dentist or staff—will remember to reinforce desirable behavior. Similarly, tasks perceived as unpleasant or of low status by the hygienist will get done by the assistant, and personal or embarrassing oversights on the part of the dentist can be caught or rectified by the hygienist. When there is open communication, they will work as a team, supporting one another.

Whether or not a complicated communication network disrupts or enhances the dental office environment depends on the commitment of each staff member to being tuned-in to the responsibilities and functions of everyone in the office.

Merely stating that communication should take place along certain pathways is not enough. The kinds of communication that should, but may or may not, actually occur will be determined by the perceptions and biases each person in the communication network brings to his/her role in the dental office.

To avoid errors, to allow treatment to proceed efficiently and comfortably, and to provide for a positive or enjoyable working environment, it is essential that roles be carefully defined and that effective communication take place along *all* possible pathways.

Defining staff roles means making it clear to each group member (1) what is expected of him/her and (2) where, when, and what types of rewards or satisfaction are possible.

The patient's participation in the functional office group is the result of the receptionist, the assistant, the hygienist, and dentist understanding how the communication process with the patient begins, what type of patient communications and other behaviors are to be positively reinforced, and how each member of the staff maintains the communication network. Practically, this understanding means:

1. The *receptionist* recognizes the patient's needs or problems and allows some patient control over appointment time, recall program, and payments. At the same time, the receptionist clearly communicates with the patient an

understanding of office policy and procedures and expected or preferred patient behaviors.

2. The *assistant* deals with possible patient anxiety in the operatory chair over upcoming procedures, checks for patient comfort, and may inform the patient about what to expect next. The assistant should expect and encourage cooperative patient behavior and should reward it by praising the patient and making appropriately timed comments to other members of the staff.

3. The *hygienist* initially accepts previous dental behaviors and attitudes towards oral hygiene even if they are inadequate. With a positive orientation, the hygienist teaches the patient proper oral hygiene, allowing the patient control, wherever possible, over the rate of learning, and appropriate skills. The hygienist maintains clear and firm communication with the patient regarding desired patient behaviors and why they are important to the dental staff as well as to the patient; the hygienist allows the patient to question office procedures and answers technical questions.

4. The *dentist* maintains leadership and control over the management of the patient's oral health but at the same time allows an appropriate degree of patient and staff freedom over treatment sequence, esthetics, choice of anesthetic, and so forth. The dentist makes certain that the patient has a clear understanding of office procedures, policies, fees, expected oral hygiene, and preventive behaviors.

5. *Group meetings* are held by the office staff. Preplanning and organization of tasks, as well as the identification of rewards and sources of satisfaction, are important considerations that must be resolved and mutually understood by the office staff *before the patient appears.* Periodic review of how satisfied the individual staff members are is essential to the maintenance of group cohesiveness and to the reinforcement of group norms. Some time each week needs to be spent in this type of group meeting.

Question: Given the opportunity to employ one dental auxiliary, which role would you wish to give up to a second person, and what functions would this person perform?

Answer: The first role most dentists wish to give up is the receptionist role, with its functions of telephone and appointment management, patient greetings, and so on. When only one auxiliary is employed, this person is often a hygienist-receptionist or a receptionist-assistant.

A certain amount of status is associated with each role. Some roles, such as that of the dentist, seem to automatically carry the most status. However, there is no necessary consistency to the so-called pecking order that may exist in a particular dental office, when it comes to who is the best communicator or who takes charge and ameliorates difficulties between staff and patients or even among the staff. As the dental staff works together, it becomes apparent that one or another of them seems to be better suited for defining the communication pathways and setting the tone for how patients and staff relate. By no means must the dentist be at the top when it comes to communication skills; the natural and democratic evolution of leadership can occur.

The natural evolution of a particular person into this role of leadership for establishing patient and staff communication has advantages and disadvantages. The advantages of a natural evolution of roles are:

1. Given the freedom, people will do what they like to do; this type of work situation enhances a sense of self-esteem and leads to job satisfaction.
2. The natural development of leadership in a group typically leads to less friction over authority and orders, since the group members do not perceive the leader as being forced on them.

Disadvantages of a natural evolution of roles are:

1. The self-perception of roles by individual group members may clash— two or more members may desire a leadership role, and each may have a different notion of how things should be done.
2. Often, what passes for natural evolution is really abdication of responsibility for defining roles carefully, so that some tasks never seem to get done. Other tasks may be performed haphazardly and inefficiently because in the particular mix of dental staff, no one likes a particular function (for example, talking about collection of late fees) or everyone assumes it is being done by someone else (for example, making the patient feel comfortable and valuable).

The dental office communication network (who starts the process of communication and who has the right to determine policy) is, therefore, shaped by:

1. The clarity of role definition
2. The perception of how leadership evolves
3. The perceived status or pecking order of the dental staff

The group dynamics existing in a group of people working together are a major determinant of the communication process among these people. Communication, cohesiveness, and conformity characterize how the members of the group relate to each other. Too often, different kinds of communication go on between the members of a group and people outside of it.

Question: Define the terms used when discussing communication by matching the definitions with the appropriate terms.

_____ A. Cohesiveness

_____ B. Conformity

_____ C. Communication network

_____ D. Group dynamics

_____ E. Functional groups

1. Who is communicating with whom; the verbal and non-verbal interactional possibilities.
2. Common goals, shared norms; mutual involvement in social interaction for a common goal.
3. Adherence to group expectancies.
4. Influential processes occurring in small face-to-face groups.
5. A sense of "we"; the forces that act on members to remain in the group.

Answer: A 5   D 4
            B 3   E 2
            C 1

24

A dentist, seated on the stool, and his assistant are laughing over an amusing incident that must have just happened, when a patient appears at the doorway. Somewhat hesitatingly, the patient makes her way between the dentist and his assistant toward the dental chair, sits down, and waits. At that moment the receptionist sticks her head in the door, says something inaudible to the patient, and the three of them (the dentist, the assistant, and the receptionist) begin laughing together. Almost absentmindedly, the dentist reaches for a mouth mirror, which the assistant has placed on the instrument tray, and still half attending to what is going on between the assistant and the receptionist, asks the patient to open her mouth. The patient, instead, asks, "But aren't you going to wash your hands, Doctor?" The laughter immediately stops. The dentist and assistant exchange embarrassed glances, and the dentist gets up and washes his hands.

Question: What does the incident cited above tell you about the group dynamics? The kinds of interactions among the members of the group in that particular setting? Indicate with a plus or minus whether each quality listed below is present or absent within the group and between the group and the patient.

	Within the group	Between the group and the patient
Cohesiveness		
Conformity		
Communication		

Answer: Clearly, a problem exists; cohesiveness, conformity, and communication are evident among the group members—the dentist, the assistant, and the receptionist—but these qualities are not evident between the group and a person outside the group—the patient.

It is very desirable to enhance the functional working group aspect of the dentist and the dental staff by:
1. Reinforcing those aspects of the group dynamics that enhance cohesiveness
2. Allowing for conformity to agreed-on norms and behaviors
3. Facilitating an open communication network
The dental office group has an element of uniqueness that is both fascinating and challenging—the role of the patient in the group. One of the characteristics of the kind of group we are discussing is, by definition, that only a small number of well-established roles (in this case, the roles of the dentist and the auxiliaries) are included.

Question: What about the patient? In your view, is the patient a member of the dental office's functional working group?

Answer: If you said, "Yes," how do you handle the problem of defining the group when the patient is not there? If you said, "No," how do you handle the problem of the patient feeling left out or like an unwelcome intruder when he/she appears for treatment?

Question: Allowing the patient's self-perception as a valued member of the dental office group to develop is a responsibility of everyone having a role in the dental treatment setting. Why is this patient self-perception so important?

Answer: The patient's self-perception of being an "in" member of the group makes it easier for the group to achieve many of its objectives, such as rendering efficient, humane care, allowing the patient to feel satisfied, and allowing the group members to feel satisfied over their performances regarding treatment, appointment, and financial requirements.

Question: How would you assign functions to the receptionist, assistant, hygienist, and dentist to enhance the development of patient self-perception?

Answer: This question can be adequately answered only through group discussion followed by role playing and further discussion.

Group dynamics can be usefully applied to overcome patient resistance to needed dental care, changing attitudes and behaviors concerning oral hygiene, and accepting and monitoring preventive dentistry programs. The process by which *group dynamics* influence individual group member behavior first requires that the involved individual feels a *cohesiveness* to the members of the group. The *communications network* can then provide *group support* for the patient *to conform* to the desired *norms* of the group, which include cooperative dental patient behaviors, behavioral modifications of oral hygiene and preventive practice, and so on. The more central to the communication network the patient can be, the more satisfied and welcome the patient is likely to feel, especially if the patient's perception is one of *accessibility* and *control* over the flow of communication.

Question: How do you get the patient to feel "in" the group?

Answer: Group leadership, when it is democratic as opposed to autocratic, fosters greater group involvement. More members of the group are likely to be task-motivated and affiliation-motivated if they have been involved in (1) determining the tasks of the group, (2) establishing norms for staff-patient behavior, and (3) creating the communication process among group members.

A certain amount of communication is inevitable in every dental treatment setting, and much of the above discussion may merely categorize what is going on anyway. It is always desirable to keep the group communication process as spontaneous as possible, allowing it to fit the personalities and needs of the individual (staff and patient) group members.

These minimal guidelines are not intended as an exhaustive list of elements in dental staff-patient communication. Hopefully, they will serve to orient and stimulate thinking concerning the responsibility and desirability of creating group dynamic processes that keep the staff and the patient comfortable with each other.

SECTION II CONDUCTING THE INTERVIEW

4 Initiating the interview

A patient may visit a dental office for a variety of reasons that range from acute illness to a routine checkup to getting advice concerning a dental problem in the family. Each of these reasons will require a different approach to the interview. This section deals primarily with diagnostic interviews; however, the techniques learned here are useful for other types of patient encounters.

OPENING STATEMENT

Question: Formulate your opening remarks for the following situation. Mrs. Arnold has been seated in your operatory by the assistant. The record indicates that Mrs. Arnold is 35 years old, the mother of three children, lives in town, was referred to you by Mrs. Jackson, and has requested this first visit because of dull pain during chewing. The assistant noted that Mrs. Arnold was anxious and concerned about her discomfort.

Answer: The opening remarks would be something like the following: Mrs. Arnold? I am . . . (your name).

The opening statement in initiating the history is important. It sets the tone of the professional relationship as well as the direction of the interview.

Question: Which of the following questions would *not* be appropriate in this situation?
A. How do you like this weather?
B. What troubles are you having?
C. I see you live in town; how long have you lived here?
D. Have you known Mrs. Jackson a long time?
E. What is the situation that brings you here today?

Answer: A, C, and D. These questions have the quality of breaking the ice, and they are used to put the patient at ease. But the question is raised as to whether a patient who is paying for your time wants to spend part of it talking about one of these topics. Another objection to these choices is that they do not set the stage for a professional relationship.

Even though you may have information about the patient, you must learn from the patient directly, why he/she has come.

Question: Which of the following openings would you choose to elicit this information from Mrs. Arnold?

A. The information I have indicates you have a dull pain during chewing. Tell me about it.
B. What troubles are you having?
C. What is the situation that brings you here today?
D. You have a dull pain during chewing?
E. How are things?

Answer: *B* and *C* give the patient freedom and define the area of discussion.

A and *D* restrict the patient's response to the topic she reported to the assistant. Frequently a patient will initially give a reason for the visit (sometimes referred to as an "admission ticket") that is a partial truth. Immediate exploration limited to the admission ticket may obscure the real reason for the visit.

E gives the patient a great deal of freedom, but it does not differentiate the interview from a social visit.

Once the patient has given information to members of the dental staff other than yourself, you need to let the patient know what you know about him/her. By stating what you know at the beginning of the interview in a frank and honest manner, you show interest in the information the patient has given and encourage a forthright relationship. The following combination of *A* and *C* is a suggested opening statement to Mrs. Arnold: "I am _____. I understand that you have a dull pain during chewing. What is the situation?"

With this opening statement Mrs. Arnold is not limited to discussing her sore jaw but is free to begin the interview in any manner she chooses. In addition, you have honestly shared and checked your information with her, allowing for immediate correction of any misunderstandings.

The receptionist indicates that Mr. Glenn has come to the office because of a broken partial denture. As he sits down, you notice that his upper partial denture is loose.

Question: Write your opening statement.

Answer: Compare your response to the following:
Mr. Glenn, I am Dr. _____. The assistant tells me that your denture is broken. What is the situation?

It is tempting to call attention to your astute observation and ask about the upper denture. This action would direct the patient's immediate response to the prosthesis, however, without giving him an opportunity to discuss another topic of perhaps greater concern. You can always ask about the upper denture later if he does not mention it.

THERAPEUTIC CONTRACTS

For every relationship between two persons there are either spoken or unspoken rules that make up the agreement or contract. The dental professional–patient relationship is no exception. In fact, there are usually three contracts established in the course of treating a patient. The dental professional and patient agree (1) to relate, (2) to exchange information, and (3) to give and receive treatment. When the staff and the patient do not agree on the terms of these contracts, the results are misleading communications, anger, and misunderstandings.

Question: You ask a patient what the trouble is, and the patient responds with, "That is what I came to you to find out." What is the implied contract?

Answer: The usual professional-patient contract is not accepted by this patient. The patient is deviating from the usual patient role by neither giving information freely nor helping you understand what is troubling him. In such a situation you must decide whether or not to accept the patient's implied contract of not giving information and continue to deal with this resistant (dependent) patient or whether the patient can be helped to modify his position. If you do not accept the contract implied by the patient in this example, you must discuss the situation with the patient and establish a contract to which both of you can agree. If a compromise cannot be reached, a last resort may be for the patient to find another dental office.

The implied contract is: "Take care of me. Don't ask me to take any responsibility for my care."

The contract of the therapeutic relationship is defined by a discussion concerning what the patient expects and wants from the relationship and what the dentist and the dental staff are able and willing to offer. (See example on p. 125.)

FACILITATIONS AND OPEN-ENDED QUESTIONS

facilitation A verbal or nonverbal communication that encourages the patient to say more, yet does not specify the area or topic to be discussed. Often, a facilitation is followed by a silence suggesting that the patient should say more.

open-ended question A question asking for information from the patient and specifying the content in general terms.*

Question: Which of the following are facilitations:
A. How are things?
B. Uh huh!
C. What troubles are you having?
D. You have been having pain in your jaw—tell me about it.

Answer: *A* and *B*
C and *D* are an open-ended question and an open-ended response that specify the area to be discussed—troubles and pain in the jaw. *C* and *D* give the patient freedom in his/her reply but differ from a facilitation by giving some structure to the answer.

---

*Blyth, J. W., and Alter, M.: How to conduct a selection interview, Los Angeles, 1965, Sherbourne Press, p. 344.

Other examples of open-ended questions are "What brings you to see me?" and "How did it happen?"

Open-ended questions and facilitations are useful for opening an interview and for following the patient's opening of a new topic. Early in the discussion of a topic, you want to know the following:

How the patient views the topic.

What the patient thinks is related, and important, to the topic.

How much the patient can tell you about the topic on his/her own before you question him/her more actively.

Question: A patient points to his lower jaw and says to you, "You know, last week I had a pain right here in my jaw." This is the first time you have heard about any symptoms related to this patient's lower jaw. What is your response?

Answer: Examples of a facilitation or open-ended questions you might have chosen are:

Uh huh! (Facilitation)

What can you recall about it? (Open-ended question)

What was it like? (Open-ended question)

Tell me about it. (Open-ended request)

In the middle of an interview another patient tells you about having some pain during eating. You want to know more about it.

Question: Write out your response to this patient. What type of response will you make?

Answer: What did you notice about it? (Open-ended question)

Silence with an expression that says, "I am interested, tell me more." (Facilitation)

5 Assisting the patient's narrative

REASSURANCE, EMPATHY, AND SUPPORT

reassurance　A response that tends to establish a sense of merit, well-being, or self-reliance in the patient.[*]

empathy　A response that recognizes or names the patient's feeling and does not in any way criticize it; the interviewer accepts the feeling in the patient even though the interviewer may believe the feeling to be wrong.

support　A response that shows interest in, concern for, or understanding of the patient.[†]

Question:　Reassurance, empathy, and support are three somewhat similar types of responses made by interviewers. All three deal with the _____ of the patient rather than with the literal meaning of what the patient is saying.

Answer:　Feelings

Each patient maintains a feeling of well-being, of being acceptable to him/herself and others, and of meeting certain standards of behavior. The manifestations of the patient's attempts to maintain a feeling of "goodness" are in opposition to divulging information that exposes his/her failures, weaknesses (as he/she views them), and inability to perform expected tasks. A feeling of being defective may interfere with the patient's ability to share openly his/her symptoms with a dental professional, who may choose to use a noncritical approach of reassurance, empathy, and support to penetrate this natural resistance or defense.

Reassurance

Reassurance can be used to decrease the patient's resistance to discussing a topic. A patient says, "I shouldn't complain about this pain, but I just can't stand the constant ache."

Question:　How do you let this patient know that you understand the severe pain she is in?

---

[*]Verwoerdt, A.: Communication with the fatally ill, Springfield, Ill., 1966, Charles C Thomas, Publisher, pp. 34-37.

[†]Enelow, A. J., and Wexler, M.: Psychiatry in the practice of medicine, New York, 1966, Oxford University Press, Inc., pp. 59-60

33

Answer: Compare your response to the following:

That pain is enough to get to anyone.

It's hard to take when there is no relief.

That kind of pain is hard to take when there is no relief. A constant pain is very disturbing. (I understand.)

A patient says, "My wife gets tired of my soft diet and every now and then fixes me something that tears up my mouth. Then I go back to taking pain killers. In a few days I get comfortable. If only I could get back to normal and not be concerned about what I eat."

Question: Make up a response showing that you understand this patient's impatience.

Answer: Compare your response to the following:

It would surely be nice to be able to enjoy some corn-on-the-cob and apples again, wouldn't it?

It really tests your patience, doesn't it?

As a member of the dental staff, you are often called on to offer reassurance (restore confidence) to the patient in panic. You give this reassurance nonverbally, by being calm yourself. Since distress and anxiety are contagious, manipulation of the physical environment of the panicky patient is used as an adjunct to reassurance. All other persons, such as relatives, are removed from the presence of the patient so that you and the patient are in a quiet office or operatory. This action reassures the patient that you do not fear the patient's loss of control, that a guard or attendant is not needed, and that you are ready to offer help.

Empathy

A patient who is having extensive dental restoration being done says, "I just can't stand it here in this chair any longer. I want out of the chair."

Question: What would be an empathic response?

Answer: Does your response recognize the feeling and show acceptance of it? The patient is restless, panicky, or irritated with having to have this treatment, with having the dental problem, and with being dependent on you to have it fixed. Compare your answer with the following:

This treatment gets to you after a few minutes.

It's no fun having this done to you and having to be dependent on someone else to get it done, is it?

Empathy, as used here, helps the patient to express his feelings more directly, dealing with them openly and without embarrassment.

It is important to realize that an empathic response does not involve giving advice or reassurance, doing something about the feeling, or even saying that the feeling is or is not justified. One merely recognizes the feeling and allows and accepts the patient's expression of it.

A patient says after a week of wearing new complete dentures, "I surely thought that I would be able to wear this set and adjust to them. I have done the best I can. I tried everything that you told me to do, but nothing seems to work."

Question: Write an emphatic response to this patient.

Answer: Does your response name the patient's feeling and accept his having it and expressing it?

Question: Which of the following is an empathic response to this patient? What is wrong with the other responses?
A. This new adhesive came in this morning's mail; let's shift over to it.
B. When you try hard and still are unable to wear the teeth, no one can blame you for being discouraged.
C. Don't be too impatient; give the teeth a little time.
D. When you can't seem to get comfortable with them, I can see how you would be discouraged.

Answer: *A* ignores the patient's feeling and gives directions or advice that would close the subject to further understanding. It also abandons the notion that the dentures are good in and of themselves.
B names and accepts the feelings, but it also provides an unnecessary justification for the feeling.
C is a mild reprimand to the patient for showing his feeling and also gives advice.
D is empathic.

A patient says, "Since I broke this tooth on the job, the company dentist saw me twice. He took some x-rays and said it was all okay. He saw me just one more time and gave me a prescription for the pain, but he didn't suggest any other treatment. I felt he wasn't doing all that he could. He wanted me to return to work and not use any of my workman's compensation. He should have really done more for me."

Question: What is a response that would empathize with the patient but not justify his feeling?

Answer: Your response might be similar to one of the following:
You felt a little unhappy with the dentist's treatment!
You felt that your tooth needed more attention?
You felt that the dentist should have done more for you?
You felt that the dentist did not show you enough concern?

Support

Supportive responses can either enhance the patient's description of his illness or close the topic to further discussion.

A patient says, "I don't know what to do when I take the medicine and get no relief. I want to go to sleep, but the pain keeps me awake, and then I just don't know what to do."

Question: Which of the following supportive responses would lead to further discussion, and which ones would close the topic?
A. It is not unusual for patient's to complain of this trouble. I know how you must feel.
B. That surely is upsetting. Such a pain upsets anyone. It will be better.
C. This is the most difficult part of your treatment. It will be better.

D. Don't be too upset about it; you will feel much better next week.

E. This is a difficult time. You feel that you need something more at night?

Answer: *A, B, C,* and *D* all tend to close the topic to further discussion. Think for a moment how you, as a patient, would respond to each.

E, on the other hand, requests the patient to continue talking about what he feels is needed.

Direct reassurance, given early in discussing a topic, tends to close the discussion. Empathy and support can be equally helpful to the patient and do not tend to close the discussion. From time to time each type of response is useful.

A patient recovering from periodontal surgery on the mandible says, "Doctor, I have been waiting for 3 days. Will I get over this and be able to eat as I did before?" You do not know what this patient has been thinking and with what he has scared himself. You want to know what his fears are. He is asking for support. You believe that he will be able to eat as before.

Question: What is a supportive response that would not close the topic to discussion?

Answer: Compare your answer to the following:

Why do you ask?

Now, what is on your mind that prompts this question?

Sounds like you have been doing a lot of thinking.

These responses are not supportive on the surface, but they show your interest in the patient, which is very supportive. A directly supportive response might be:

Yes, but you seem to be having some doubts?

CONFRONTATIONS

confrontation A response that points out to the patient his/her feeling, behavior, or previous statement.*

Confrontations are most effective in focusing the patient's attention on his/her feeling, behavior, or statement. They may also let the patient know you understand what he/she said. Many times you may make a special inflection or insinuation in repeating the patient's statement to emphasize a part of it.

Question: Which of the following could be considered confrontations?

A. You look unhappy.

B. When I touch this tooth, you grimace.

C. You are saying the other dentists didn't understand how much trouble you are having?

D. Where did you say the pain is?

Answer: *A, B,* and *C* could be considered confrontations.

D merely asks for a point of information that you missed.

---

*Enelow, A. J., and Wexler, M.: Psychiatry in the practice of medicine, New York, 1966, Oxford University Press, Inc., pp. 59-60.

You learn from a patient who has intermittent temperomandibular joint pain that he had a bad attack last Saturday. He said that nothing happened to cause the attack. You then get him to tell you about Saturday, and he says, "After about 1 hour of work at the office I went to the airport to pick up my father-in-law. We went to lunch and then home with the family. That afternoon we sat around and talked. I first noticed the pain at lunch." You know from previous information that his father-in-law owns the business he operates, so you want to focus on the fact that his father-in-law came to town.

Question: What is your response?

Answer: The following are several examples of confrontations:
You met your father-in-law at the airport?
Nothing happened Saturday to cause an attack, but you did meet your father-in-law at the airport?
Your father-in-law came to town Saturday?

A patient complains to you, "The treatments you are giving me are costing too much." You sense that the patient wants you to change the treatment.

Question: What is your response?

Answer: Compare your response with the following:
You sound like you want me to change your treatment.
Too much? Is the price really a problem?
You seem to be complaining about the treatment.

A young patient tells you, "My father feels I am taking too much medicine for this pain." As the patient tells you this, you notice that his fist clenches. You wish to focus his attention on your observation.

Question: Make up a response that will confront this patient with his behavior.

Answer: Compare your response with the following:
Were you aware you clenched your fist when you spoke of your father's feeling?
You said that with a clenched fist!

REFLECTIONS

reflection A response that repeats, mirrors, or echoes a portion of what the patient just said.

Although it focuses on a particular point, a reflection helps the patient to continue in his/her own style.

Question: Which of the following might be reflections?
A. And then?
B. It hurt?
C. You could not eat?
D. Nervous?

Answer: *B, C,* and *D*
A would be a reflection if the patient had said, "and then . . ." without completing the sentence. Otherwise it is considered an open-ended question.

A patient says, "I have had a pain in this upper tooth for 3 weeks. Then last Saturday I noticed that it had spread up around my eye . . . "

Question: Reflect this statement and focus the patient on the spread of the pain so that the patient can continue.

Answer: Around your eye?

To avoid miscommunication, it is best to use the exact words the patient used.

A patient says, "The pain was worse last night. It was really bad."

Question: Reflect this statement to the patient to learn what she means by "bad."

Answer: You might focus the patient's attention on "bad" by asking:
Bad?
It was bad?
The pain was worse?

Note the use of the patient's exact words.

INTERPRETATIONS

interpretation A confrontation that is based on an inference rather than an observation.*

An interpretation usually links events or ascribes motives or feeling to the patient's reply or behavior.

Question: Which of the following might be considered an interpretation? Which is a confrontation?
A. You seem unhappy.
B. You upset me.
C. You just clenched your fist.
D. Sounds like you do not like the assistant.
E. You reacted the same way when your wisdom tooth was extracted.

Answer: A, D, and E are interpretations.
B and C report your unaltered observation of the patient and of your own reaction and are thus confrontations.

A patient says, "When I went into the supervisor's office this morning, this pain in my tooth was really bad." You learned earlier that same thing had occurred on a previous visit to the supervisor's office and that even as a child going to her father's study, this patient would have increased discomfort from aches and pains.

Question: Interpret this information to the patient, making an inference concerning the association or cause. Then make up a confrontation response to the patient.

---

*Blyth, J. M., and Alter, M.: How to conduct a selection interview, Los Angeles, 1965, Sherbourne Press, p. 357. Enelow, A. J., and Wexler, M.: Psychiatry in the practice of medicine, New York, 1966, Oxford University Pres, Inc., pp. 59-60.

Compare your responses with the following:

Interpretation:

Sounds like seeing the supervisor now was like seeing your father when you were a child. Both make your pains worse.

Confrontation:

Just when you went in?

Into the supervisor's office?

Your pain became worse?

Just by going into the supervisor's office?

SILENCE

silence A communication, a response.

Those scientists who study communication report that *we cannot fail to communicate*. A silence can show interest or lack of interest; it can also show support or withdrawal. Most useful to the dentist are the supportive silence and the interested silence.

A patient says, "I'm unhappy about the way this new cap looks." You want the patient to tell you more about his feelings toward the appearance of the cap.

Question: How might you respond?

A. Uh huh.

B. Silence (while you look at the patient's record or at your instrument tray).

C. Silence (while you nod "yes").

D. Silence (while you relax and shift back into your chair).

E. Silence (while you shift forward in your chair with increased attention).

Answer: *A*, *C*, and *E* show interest and support in what the patient is saying. This interest and support should encourage further discussion of the topic.

B is usually interpreted by patients as a withdrawal from them, lack of interest, or both.

D may be interpreted as a withdrawal from the patient or as "Now I am relaxed and ready to really listen."

The patient interprets your silence positively when you focus your attention on the patient and away from objects on the tray or table next to you.

Patients frequently come to the dental office with the idea or an assumed contract that they are in the interview only to answer specific questions. To counter this belief, silence early in the interview may make the interchange much more productive and could make your job as interviewer much easier.

Interviewer: What troubles are you having?

Patient: My gums have been bleeding. (Pause—waiting for your next question.)

Question: How would you respond to this patient? If you would use silence, describe your nonverbal behavior.

Answer: Silence, accompanied by nodding your head, looking at the

39

patient expectantly, or shifting your body toward the patient, might be used as a response.

Silence used too much may be interpreted by the patient to mean that the interviewer cannot think of anything to say. The patient must feel the responsibility for breaking the silence. If he/she does not feel this responsibility, silence is usually an ineffective facilitation. Silence is frequently ineffective with young teenagers, since they do not feel compelled to filled the void.

Question: If a patient were to begin crying while describing a severely frightening sensation, how would he/she react to a response of supportive, interested silence?

Answer: The patient would probably react positively, gain composure, and be able to continue the interview. Most patients feel that, somehow, the interviewer understands them and is able to accept them. Silence here shows acceptance of the act of crying.

Question: How would this crying patient react to firm reassurance that things will be better, such as, "Now, that's all right, you will feel better"?

Answer: The patient might feel guilty about making you feel uncomfortable. When the dental professional actively reassures them, many patients feel that they have done something wrong in crying.

Question: How would this same patient react to a specific question for information, such as, "What did you do to get more comfortable?"

Answer: This type of response would usually make the patient feel weak and silly for crying and that crying was not accepted in the office. However, this question might be appropriate after a period of silence during which the patient regained his/her composure. The timing of the question is all-important.

Question: How would this patient react to silence accompanied by some bodily contact, such as grasping his/her hand or placing your hand on his/her nearest shoulder?

Answer: The patient's reaction would depend on his/her interpretation of your behavior. Your behavior might be interpreted as appropriate parental concern or supportive human understanding. On the other hand, it could be interpreted either as inappropriate seductiveness or as active reassurance, which would tend to block further emotional display.

A patient's acceptance of, and reaction to, physical contact will depend on a number of variables: how the physical contact is made, the age differential between the patient and the professional, the sex of each, and the timing of the action. The timing is important with respect to the length of the professional-client relationship and with respect to the amount of time passing after the crying begins and before the physical contact is made.

In an interview situation the point to remember is that physical contact is interpreted on the basis of cultural expectancies that are preconscious (they are unconscious but can readily be brought into consciousness). The saying "the message is in the receiver" has special significance in this situation. Your best-intentioned touch may be misinterpreted. If you are not sure what the patient's expectancies are, it is best not to make a physical contact. The rule is, if you sense any hesitation in yourself or the patient, *do not touch*.

Another aspect of the use of silence may be brought out by the following dialogue:

> *Interviewer:* When did you first notice the pain?
>
> *Patient:* Let's see (pause), first I noticed the pain in this upper tooth last August (pause). No, it was while I was away at summer school. It was about (pause) the middle of July (pause).
>
> **Question:** How would you respond to this patient, a college student?
>
> **Answer:** This patient is having some difficulty remembering the history of his pain and needs some time to collect his thoughts. Silence on your part could be very supportive, but silence beyond 10 seconds would not be appropriate in this situation.
>
> **Question:** If, after 15 seconds, the patient remained silent, how would you respond?
>
> **Answer:** Compare your response with the following:
> What was it like then?
>
> Once the time of the onset of the present problem is established, the quality of the symptoms and the associated events at that time are the next logical pieces of information to obtain.

SUMMATIONS

> **summation** A response of an interviewer that reviews information given by the patient.

A summation response may fulfill any one of several purposes: it demonstrates the interviewer's interest in the patient's history, and it lets the patient know exactly how the interviewer interprets what the patient has presented. By summation the patient's history may be clarified. One technique of summation consists of restating what the patient related, with reemphasis. Through reemphasis the interviewer can express such ideas as, "Is this what you [the patient] really intended to say?" or "I am interested in this particular aspect of what you said; let's explore this further." A summation may also be used to bridge a change of topic.

The following are examples of summation responses:

Now, as I understand you, the pain *is* worse after meals and you never have pain at night. (This response presents the interviewer's understanding and clarifies the history.)

Do I understand you to say that you have *never* had any trouble before the episode last week? (This response questions, for clarification, what the patient has said.)

Let me review. You said that just as you bit down, you noticed a sharp pain?

(This response asks whether the patient said what he/she had intended to say.)

Let's see, the first tooth extraction was in 1963 and the next one was in 1965? (This response focuses attention on 1965 and bridges a change of topic from 1963 to 1965.)

A 27-year old mother of two children and the wife of a graduate student tells of her dental history. She says, "I have a tooth that is sensitive to hot and cold water. It feels like the tooth that was filled 8 years ago, when Dennis was born. Dr. Shaw put in an amalgam filling at that time, and I haven't had any trouble with it until last week, when I had severe pain when I took a drink at a party."

Question: Make up a separate summation responses to do each of the following:
A. Clarify the history
B. Question the patient's account
C. Focus attention on one aspect of the history

Answer: A. *Clarify the history:* The tooth was filled after your first pregnancy?
B. *Question the patient's account:* Dr. Shaw put in an amalgam filling?
C. *Focus attention on one aspect of the history:* The tooth is the same one that was filled!

All of these answers focus attention to an aspect of the history and, in part, question what the patient has said.

6 Obtaining specific information

LAUNDRY-LIST QUESTIONS

Frequently a patient will reply to a facilitation or an open-ended question with the question, "How do you mean?" The following exchange is an example.

Interviewer:	Tell me about your toothache.
Mr. Adams:	It just hurts.
Interviewer:	It hurts?
Mr. Adams:	Yes!
Interviewer:	Tell me about it.
Mr. Adams:	How do you mean?

The interviewer has now used a reflection and two open-ended requests without getting a description of the pain. At this point Mr. Adams needs some support and guidance. A technique frequently used in this situation is a *laundry-list question that gives the patient a number of alternative adjectives or descriptive phrases to use.*

Question:	Which of the following might be considered a laundry-list question? A. Is it a burning pain? B. Does the pain go up over your head? C. Does the pain feel like a burn, an ache, drawing, pressure, or piercing? D. Does the pain come on every week, every hour, every month, or every few minutes?
Answer:	*C* and *D*
Patient:	This pain is worse.
Interviewer:	How is that?
Patient:	What do you mean?
Question:	How would you phrase a laundry-list question to learn what the patient means by "worse"?

Answer: Compare your answer with the following:
Well, it is more frequent, deeper, making your whole jaw ache, keeping you awake, or what?

Question: What would be wrong with a laundry-list question such as "Do you have these pains every hour, day, or week?"

Answer: There are two possible errors in this question:
1. The patient is reluctant to give an answer that falls outside the range of frequencies that have been suggested. The above question sets the limits from 1 hour to 1 week. The patient may hesitate to answer that he is having pains every 20 minutes.
2. Since the order of frequency given in the question falls into a logical sequence, it usually gives some hint to the patient of what you expect the answer to be. Many times it is the voice inflection that gives away the expected answer.

To avoid suggesting the answer, the rule in formulating a laundry-list question is to scramble the logical sequence of items and to give limits beyond those that any patient would be expected to anwer.

Question: If a patient were having attacks of pain and you wanted to know how frequent they were, how would you phrase a laundry-list question? (Usual frequency is from one attack a day to one every 2 or 3 days.)

Answer: Compare your answer to the following, which limits but illustrates the technique:
Do you have attacks once a week, once an hour, once a month, once every 5 minutes, or once a year?

A modification of the laundry-list question can be used to draw out a patient to tell you more. When the list is limited to two items, both of which are absurd, the patient must then clarify his position.

Question: Which of the following examples would draw out the patient?
A. Is your pain just barely annoying, or has it stopped you from working?
B. I don't understand, does your pain make you vomit or can you ignore it and continue what you are doing?

Answer: Both. A pain is more than annoying if the patient is coming to the dental office about it, and most pains do not cause one to stop working or to vomit.

DIRECT QUESTIONS

direct question A response that asks for a specific bit of information.*

---

*Enelow, A. J., and Wexler, M.: Psychiatry in the practice of medicine, New York, 1966, Oxford University Press, Inc., p. 57.

A direct question can usually be answered in one word or a brief phrase.

In the opening dialogue Mr. Adams was not able to give a description of the toothache, even with the aid of open-ended questions and facilitations.

Question: What would be wrong with using one of the following questions after Mr. Adams mentioned his toothache?
Did it keep you awake at night?
Is it a throbbing pain?
Does the pain seem to be in one tooth?

Answer: Some of the faults with these questions are as follows:
1. You would be asking for a "yes" or "no" from the patient, either of which would yield little information.
2. You would be giving the patient some information as to what you thought the pain might be like or (as he would see it) what the pain *should* be like.
3. From these questions you would get confirmation or denial of your own concept of the patient's pain, not his candid description.
4. You would be encouraging an authoritarian-submissive or parent-child relationship with the patient.
5. The burden of interpreting the meaning of the questions would be placed on the patient. Since you would not be sure what his interpretation was, you would not be sure what his answer meant.

Direct questions that can be answered with one word add little information to what you already know about the patient. On the other hand, they may provide that crucial bit of information that is diagnostic.

Question: Which of the following questions would result in more information?
A. Is it a burning pain?
B. What is the pain like?
C. What seems to aggravate your toothache?
D. Does hot or cold food make your toothache worse?

Answer: *B* and *C*
A and *D* yield a very specific bit of information and could be answered by a "yes" or "no."

We do not wish to advocate avoiding all questions with one-word answers. At times such questions are most appropriate, but these times are few. After a patient has given you a description of his/her toothache that fits the symptoms of an abscess, for example, you need to know if the patient has ever had any discharge from the area.

Question: Which of the following would you ask?
A. What have you noticed in the area of the toothache?
B. Have you had any pus or a bad taste from the area of the toothache?
C. What changes have you noticed in the area of the toothache?

Answer: *B* will give you the information that you desire and will save valuable interview time. The direct question can also be used to focus a rambling patient on the topic of concern.

PROBING

In telling their symptoms, patients do not always give you all the details you need. Once they have told you about a phase of the illness, it may be necessary to probe for more specific information.

Question: Which of the following would probe for more detailed information?
A. And then?
B. What else did you notice at the time?
C. Mm hmmmm.

Answer: *A* and *B*
C would allow the patient to change the subject or proceed in any direction.

A patient has told you that she sometimes has pain near her ear after lunch. It lasts about half an hour.

Question: You want to know if there are specific foods associated with the pain. Which of the following would you ask to obtain this information?
A. What do you notice about the days when you have the pain?
B. Is there something different about the consistency or hardness of the food you eat on the days when you have the pain?
C. Do you avoid certain foods to prevent the pain?
D. Do you eat the same thing every day at lunch?
E. Tell me more about this.

Answer: *B*, *C*, and *D*
A and *E* would allow the patient to wander too far from the information that you want.

A patient tells you about a toothache that is worse in the morning and after a day during which he was tense and smoked more than usual. He tells you about its frequency and persistence and about the pains associated with it. You observe an intraoral swelling. You want to know whether the patient spits out pus or blood.

Question: Phrase a probing question that does not give away the answer or frighten the patient.

Answer: Compare your answer with the following:
What does your saliva look like?
What does your saliva taste like?
Has the taste of your saliva changed?
What does the saliva that you spit out look like?

Before you get the final answer on whether the patient is spitting out blood or pus, you may have to follow up these questions with an additional question, such as "Are there any red streaks in the saliva?"

CHANGING THE TOPIC

An interview is created from a number of merging topics. The dental professional guides and directs the selection of topics through many of the techniques discussed earlier and by deliberately changing (or preventing the patient from changing) the topic.

A patient has given you a very complete description of his present symptoms of a possibly genetic defect. You wish to learn if anyone in his family had similar symptoms. You want to change the topic and focus on the family.

Question: Which of the following do you prefer?
A. Does anyone in your family have similar symptoms?
B. Do you know anyone with similar problems?
C. I would like to know about your family. Does anyone in your family have similar symptoms?

Answer: *A* implies that the symptoms are caused by something in the family.
B is too open ended, since the patient is free to talk about friends and co-workers. Also, it does not prepare the patient for a change in topic.
C is preferred because it gives the patient a reason for the question. He is not left to guess why you changed the subject. From *C* the patient may well infer that you are just being thorough and avoiding the use of diagnostic terms.

When you change the subject, it is a good practice to let the patient know why; otherwise, his inferences may get in the way of treatment. If there is no logical bridge from one topic to the next, say so. Be honest with the patient. If there is a logical bridge, give it. By your concerned frankness and honesty, you will encourage the patient to be frank and honest with you.

Question: What is wrong with this exchange?

Patient: Well, I guess that's the entire story of my case of venereal sores in my mouth. I should have come in sooner.

Interviewer: How is your mother's health?

Answer: Since the interviewer did not present a logical association, the patient might well reply, "Now, what kind of a question is that? My mother doesn't have anything to do with my illness."

Question: How could the interviewer have asked the question to obtain the needed information as a logical sequence?

Answer: Compare your answer to the following:
That may be true, but we can still help you. Now, let me review the health of your family. How is your mother's health?

Interviewer:	What seems to be the trouble?
Patient:	I have had this pain for some time now. It's getting worse. Last night I hardly slept at all because of it.
Interviewer:	What's it like?
Patient:	It feels like it's down here in the middle of my jaw. Then the side of my head gets sore, and I just can't get comfortable. All of this makes my headache worse, and it begins to pound.
Question:	You want to focus on the tooth pain and come back to the headache later. What is your response?
Answer:	Does your answer let the patient know that you plan to come back to the headache? Compare your response with the following: I need more information about the tooth pain first, and then we can come back to your headache. You mentioned that you have had the pain for some time. (Pause and wait for the patient to say more about it.)

7 Specific interview problems

QUESTIONS THAT ANTAGONIZE

"From the looks of your mouth, you have not been brushing as we instructed you. Why aren't you taking care of your teeth?"

Question: What is wrong with this question?

Answer: This question antagnoizes the patient, accuses him of wrong-doing, and tends to put him on the defensive. If you put a patient on the defensive, he will probably say very little and will not be encouraged to cooperate with you and tell the truth.

Question: If the patient were at ease with you, he would speak _____, and you would obtain a much more reliable history.

Answer: Freely

Each of the following word pairs contains an emotionally neutral word and an emotionally charged word.

Question: Select the emotionally neutral word from each pair:
A. Cancer-Growth
B. Unsatisfactory-Bad
C. Upset-Mad
D. Blood colored-Reddish
E. Doesn't care-Casual
F. Inform-Complain
G. Order-Ask
H. Yellow-Jaundiced

Answer: A. Growth
B. Unsatisfactory
C. Upset
D. Reddish
E. Casual
F. Inform
G. Ask
H. Yellow

Question: Select the question in each pair that is less provoking of defensiveness:

A. Why did you stop eating?
B. What was it that made eating solid foods impossible?

C. Did you think you had a growth?
D. Did you think you had a cancer?

E. That must have made you mad.
F. That must have upset you.

G. Did you give in to the pain?
H. Did the pain force you to stop what you were doing?

I. How long have you treated this yourself before coming in?
J. How long have you suffered with this?

Answer: *B, C, F, H,* and *J*

Question: Rephrase the following so that the emotionally loaded connotations, which may antagonize, are taken out:

A. Did you follow my directions in taking the medicine?
B. Why did you quit brushing your teeth?
C. Why did you wait until tonight to see about this?
D. Now, just tell me about your tooth without all of the other information.

Answer: Compare your responses with the following:

A. How are you taking your medicine now?
B. What caused you to stop brushing your teeth?
C. Were you able to see about this earlier?
D. Let's just focus on your tooth so that I can understand what you are experiencing.

The real world is rarely divided into black and white, all or nothing. It is made up of shades or degrees of a quality, sensation, or feeling. A dental professional's questions need to take this into account and ask for the degree of a sensation rather than for a choice between the extremes. More information will come forth if it is sought in terms of degrees rather than absolutes.

Question: Choose the question that will obtain more information:

A. Do you have difficulty chewing solid foods?
B. What foods are you able to eat?

Answer: *B*

To *A* the patient may reply with "yes" or "no" and feel no pressure to say more. In reality the patient may be having some trouble chewing solids, but from your question may not think that it is enough difficulty to justify a "yes" reply. In this situation the patient decides where to draw the line between "no difficulty" and "difficulty" and answers accordingly. With *B* you obtain the information from the patient and then you decide whether the patient's difficulties fit into your category of "no difficulty" or "difficulty." You take responsibility for judging the significance of the patient's experience.

Question: Select the question in each pair that obtains more specific information and underscore the phrase that makes it so:

A. Is it possible that you were at fault when you were injured?

B. Is it possible that you were partially at fault when you were injured?

C. Have you had sore gums?

D. Have you had more than usual soreness in your gums?

E. Do you have headaches that are not relieved by aspirin?

F. Do you have headaches?

Answer: *B, partially*

D, more than usual soreness

E, that are not relieved by aspirin

We have considered questions that may antagonize a patient because they accuse the patient of wrongdoing or because they scare the patient with an emotionally loaded word. We have also considered questions that call on the patient to decide whether the degree of a quality is sufficient in the patient's experience to justify a "yes" answer. Finally, we have considered questions that vary in the degree of specificity in which they direct the patient to answer. In regard to the last pairs of questions presented, the broader, less specific question is usually more appropriate when a topic is being opened, whereas the more specific question is usually more appropriate in the later discussion of a topic. When you are opening a topic, your intent is to gather as much data as quickly as possible. Thus, general questions and facilitations are used. Later in the discussion you are ready to wrap up the topic and pull in missing bits of information, and more specific questions are appropriate. The key point is that you must be in control and aware of what you are doing. With practice you can precisely direct an interview in its gentleness, lack of antagonism, degree of specificity, and degree of comfort for the patient.

There are times when the situation warrants the risk and your rapport is sufficient to allow you to provoke, confront aggressively, and be blunt with the patient. These procedures are sometimes indicated to move the passive or dependent patient, to convince the patient that he/she needs to modify his/her behavior, and to convince the patient that you care enough to risk losing his/her good feelings toward you or to risk losing him/her as a patient. Just know what you are doing and why you are doing it; know when you want to be warm, friendly, and compassionate and when you want to be difficult, confronting, and direct. There are times when each style is appropriate and constructive for patient growth and acceptance of increased responsibility.

Introductory and softening phrases are useful when you are obtaining social and personal information from the patient.

Question: Modify the following questions to make them more acceptable to the patient:

A. Did the situation anger you?

B. Was it your fault that you got hit in the mouth?

C. Were you unhappy with your previous dentist?

D. Do you get irritated with dentists who do not follow your requests?

Answer: Compare your answers with the following:
    A. Would you say that the situation tended to anger you?
    B. Do you feel that it was partially your fault that he hit you in the mouth?
    C. Is it possible that you were unhappy with your previous dentist?
    D. Would you be willing to say that dentists who do not follow your requests annoy you?

"YES" OR "NO" ANSWERS

With some patients there is a danger in using questions requiring "yes" or "no" answers. The patient's answer may be more dependent on the immediate milieu than on the facts.

When a question is answered with a "yes," you cannot be sure what the "yes" means. Is it given to please you, to give you what the patient thinks you want to hear, or to avoid discussing an area that the patient wants to avoid, or is it a factual response? The following questions might be answered with a "yes" for any of the above reasons:

Have you been able to take the medicine?
You saw a dentist about that trouble 3 years ago?
Are you getting along all right with your job now?
Are you able to stay on the diet?

When a question is answered with a "no," the same situation arises as with questions that are answered with a "yes."

Question: The patient may just wish to disagree, to _____, or to _____ discussing the topic, or the patient may be giving a _____ response.

Answer: Please, avoid, factual

Several examples of questions that will yield "no" answers of ambiguous meaning are as follows:

Have you had any trouble with your ears?
Do you take sedatives frequently?
Did you have trouble with the false teeth?
Have you been sick before?
Have you had sick headaches?
Do you eat excessively?
Do you kick your dog?
Do you scream at your children?

"WHY" QUESTIONS

Question: What is wrong with questions such as "Why did you take that medicine?" or "Why did you take out your denture?" or "Why didn't you wear your retainer?"

Answer: These questions call on the patient to account for his/her behavior. Since much of the patient's behavior may be unconscious or related to reasons that are not socially acceptable, the patient may be antagonized by the inference in the question. The patient may feel that such a question finds fault with him/her and may thus become irritated or annoyed. It is difficult to begin a question with "why" and avoid the overtones of accusation. In addition, "why" questions come from a whining position on the part of the person asking the question. The whining position may be described as a position of helplessness, pleading, or angry frustration. The next time you ask a "why" question, stop and check whether one of these feelings applies to you.

Question: What is wrong with questions such as "Why did you have a toothache Saturday afternoon?" or "Why were you so tense this morning with the discomfort?"

Answer: If the patient knew why he/she felt the way he/she did, the patient would understand his/her illness and might not need your services. In addition, the patient's usual response to one of these questions will be a rationalization.

The answer to a "why" question is a "because." Since we are not always capable of understanding our own behavior, the "because" answer is often the most socially acceptable answer we can come up with. It is an alibi, an excuse, or in professional terms, a rationalization. Rationalizations are of interest to some but are of little or no value in the professional interview or interaction.

An alternative to asking "why?" is to make an honest statement to the patient, such as "It is not clear . . . " or "I do not understand the situation. Tell me more about how you see it." Such responses will not irritate or antagonize the patient. They show interest and are supportive. They may produce a rationalization, but the patient generally does not feel as defensive as he would with a direct, whining "why" question.

SUGGESTIVE QUESTIONS

Interviewer: When you discussed your problem, your breathing was a little rapid. Were you at ease, or were you a little nervous?

Patient: I was a little nervous.

Question: What was wrong with the interviewer's question?

Answer: The interviewer gave the patient the answer as well as the question. To avoid this error, the interviewer could have asked, "What was the situation when you discussed your dental problem?" The interviewer could then later have asked, "Were you at ease?"

To varying degrees, both the experienced interviewer and the novice ask questions that suggest the answers.

Question: Rephrase the following questions so that they do not suggest the answers.
A. Has the pain gone to the top of your head?
B. Is the pain worse during eating?
C. Some patients report nausea with this medicine; does it affect you in this way?
D. May I assume that you have taken the medicine as directed?
E. Before taking the medicine do you always try to relieve the pain by relaxing your jaw?

Answer: Compare your rephrased questions with the following:
  A. Is the pain only about your tooth or do you notice it elsewhere?
  B. What is the pain like after a big meal?
  C. Do you have any complaints about the medicine?
  D. How are you taking the medicine now?
  E. What do you do to relieve the pain?

One way to test a question as to whether it is a giveaway is to see if you can anticipate the answer.

Question: In which of the following can you anticipate the answer:
  A. You take the medicine after every meal, don't you?
  B. Are you able to take the medicine after every meal?

Answer: *A*
  B gives the patient an acceptable out for not following the medication directions to the letter. The patient might say that he/she is unable to take the medicine at work.

You are interviewing a patient who has been injured on the job. You want to know whether the pain in his jaw goes into his neck.

Question: Rephrase the following question to remove the suggestion that the pain might be expected to go into the patient's neck:
  Does the pain ever shoot down into your neck?

Answer: Is the pain only in your jaw?
  Do you notice the pain anywhere else?

PATIENT QUESTIONS

Patients ask questions for many different reasons. When a patient asks a question during data gathering, the patient is rarely asking for information. These questions are usually designed for other reasons. The reason for the question is not always clear.

Question: How would you respond to "Are you married? Do you have any children?"
  A. If the patient seemed to be asking a simple question for information
  B. If the patient seemed to be trying to manipulate the professional relationship

Answer: A. A simple, direct, honest reply of "yes" or "no" would be appropriate. We assume that the patient wishes to know you, the dental professional, as a real person rather than as an idealized role image. If you were correct in your assumption that the patient was just asking for information, the topic will change.
  B. "Why do you ask?" if done noncombatively, is always a safe answer. We assume in this case that the patient is asking the question to modify the professional relationship toward one that is closer, informal, and social. Should you respond "yes," you invite a more personal question, such as "Is your wife/husband happy?" or "Does your husband/wife feel lucky to have you?" These questions may lead to a nonprofessional

relationship problem. Prevent this problem before it occurs. After all, you are holding the patient's head in your arm with your head very close to his/her head. Socially, you would be considered familiar, fresh, or provocative if you initiated such a position.

The rule is to answer a patient's personal questions honestly and directly *only* when you understand clearly why they are being asked and when you are confident that your reply will further the maintenance of a comfortable professional relationship.

Question: How would you respond to questions such as "Are you a Democrat?" or "Are you a Baptist?"

Answer: These questions are generally inappropriate for a patient to ask. Your response should indicate that discussion of these topics does not contribute to the patient's care. Compare your answers to the following:
It is interesting that you ask that, but what I need to know is . . .
Why do you ask?
I don't understand how that will make a difference in my helping you.

Question: If a patient replied, "Oh, I was just wondering how you were going to vote," how would you respond?

Answer: Compare your response with the following:
I don't see how that information will help us get your problem solved.

Question: Knowing that the patient has cancer, how would you respond to "Doctor, do I have cancer?"

Answer: "Cancer" is a word that is emotionally loaded and that has, medically speaking, lost its dictionary meaning. Thus, you cannot answer the question with a simple sentence. As illustrated in the drawing, what the patient has in his head when he thinks about the word "cancer" is quite different from what the dentist has in his head when he thinks about the word "cancer."

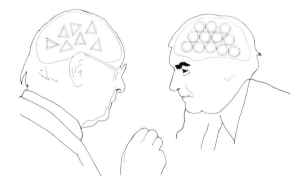

"Doctor, do I have cancer?"

You must answer the question by discussing for 5 to 10 minutes what the patient has been thinking about and what he really wants to know. An answer such as the following might initiate this discussion:

I don't know what you mean by "cancer," but maybe we can discuss exactly what you do have. Let's start with what you have been thinking about and whatever questions you have.

The response "Why do you ask?" may work very well in this situation, but it does have a gently discouraging quality to it and may offend a sensitive patient, when that is not your intention.

Question: How would you respond to "Should I continue to take both medicines?"
A. If the patient seemed to be asking a simple question for information
B. If the patient seemed to be complaining about having to take so much medicine

Answer: A. "Yes" or "no". There are situations and questions to which direct answers are indicated. Nevertheless, giving direct answers in professional interviews is the exception, not the rule.
B. "What is your feeling about the medicine?" or "Do you want to continue taking both medicines?" Since the patient decides at home whether to take the medicine, bringing his/her feelings about the medicine out into the open may make the difference between successful and unsuccessful management of the patient.

The reason many patients ask a question is not to obtain an answer but rather to direct discussion to the topic introduced by the question, to avoid the current topic, or to direct and take more control of the interaction. Rarely does the initial question cover what the patient really wants to know. As in the question about cancer, the patient wants to know specifics of what he/she can expect, rather than the general information that would be obtained by a "yes" or "no" answer.

INFORMING OF ILLNESS

Question: You have just received the pathologic confirmation that Mr. Lewis, a patient under your care, has a basal cell carcinoma. How will you inform the patient or a relative of the illness?

Answer: The following is one approach: Ask the patient, "How are you feeling now?" Obtain the patient's reply. Follow up the patient's reply by asking, "What is your understanding of what is wrong with you?" It is best to start with what the patient knows about the illness, since you may not have a clear idea of what the patient knows or fears.

Question: After learning what the patient's concept of his illness is, how will you advise him of the true nature of the illness?

Answer: One way is to give the patient the medical diagnosis and then interpret it. For example, you might say, "Mr. Lewis, we have received the report from the pathologist on the tissue removed from your mouth this week. The diagnosis is basal cell carcinoma. What do you know about this disease?"

Question: If Mr. Lewis replies, "I've never heard of that before," what will you say?

Answer: You might ask, "What questions do you have about it?" It is best to begin with information that the patient wants to know rather than with information that the patient does not want, cannot handle intellectually or emotionally, or will not hear for a variety of reasons. The patient's concerns are usually whether or not he/she will live, be able to return to work, have pain, or need surgery. If surgery is needed, the patient wants to know if it will be disfiguring.

A part of helping the patient learn about his/her illness is to get the patient to answer his/her own questions by asking, "What do you think?" and then correcting the answers. The patient may ask specific questions, to which it is best to answer as honestly as you can, keeping in mind that you never want to destroy the patient's defenses. Remember, you are helping the patient learn about his/her disease; you are not showing off how much you know. What the patient ends up knowing is the important thing, not how good you looked in the process. You want to let the patient know that regardless of what he/she is to go through, you will be supportive.

Remember, the most important part of a message is that part heard by the receiver. In this situation you are imparting information to the patient. The most important part of the process is learning what the patient hears.

Question: After you have answered the patient's questions and discussed the patient's illness, what will you say before you close the conversation?

Answer: Compare your answer to the following:
I'm concerned that we have a common understanding of your situation. Let's review how you see it now.

You will be amazed how frequently the patient's understanding is in error. If possible, you should correct the patient's misconceptions. This may not be possible when the patient has some personal need to misunderstand, such as a need to deny any imperfection in him/herself. When such a block to understanding occurs, note it and leave the resolution for a time when the patient is more receptive.

Question: How will you close the discussion?

Answer: Compare your answer to the following:
You may have further questions by your next visit. If so, please ask them. I will see you again at your next appointment, and we will discuss your questions at that time.

In caring for a patient with an illness that will persist for some time or for one who will need further therapy, it is important to encourage the patient to ask questions. This will help the patient to avoid worry. The patient who does not ask questions and clarify his/her ideas may develop a delusion about what is going on in his/her body. Such a delusion may prevent or interfere with treatment.

The patient will obviously be anxious and have many worrisome thoughts about what the future holds for him/her. When the patient is anxious, he/she often cannot clearly understand instructions about control of bleeding, taking of medications, and so on, even after routine procedures, such as tooth extractions. It is a good procedure to check out what the patient has heard you say, what he/she understands, and how he/she will handle bleeding, pain, or other predictable reactions to the procedure just completed. The process of giving instructions is similar to the process of informing the patient of a serious illness. Use the same follow-up and checking techniques, and you will have fewer calls outside of office hours.

In summary, the steps for informing a patient or a patient's relative of an illness are:

1. Find out what the patient or relative thinks or knows about the illness.
2. Find out what the patient or relative wants to know about the illness.
3. Give honest answers to the questions in such a way that you leave the patient or relative with a realistic hope.
4. Before you close the conversation, determine the patient or relative's understanding of what you have discussed.
5. Leave the communication channel open so that the patient or relative can ask further questions.

For the specific situation of having to inform a patient of a fatal illness, we suggest that you review *Communication with the Fatally Ill* by Adriaan Verwoerdt, M.D., Chapters 3 and 4.*

INTERVIEWING TRAPS

There are a number of common traps into which the beginning, and even at times the experienced interviewer, falls. Many of these traps are covered in earlier discussions of specific techniques to be used in conducting the interview.

The question that can be answered with a "yes" or "no" is fraught with miscommunications. Reasons for the patient responding with a "yes" or "no" may range from giving factual information to wanting to please or displease you. The patient may even be trying to avoid further discussion of the topic or hasten the end of the interview.

Suggestive questions give the patient the answer to the question or at least let the patient know the answer that you are seeking. With the patient who has a need to please others, this answer will probably be what you expected to hear.

Multiple questions have one specific use and many difficulties. The one specific use is to encourage a quiet patient to take responsibility and talk more freely. By asking multiple questions, the patient (if he/she can remember all of the questions) is encouraged to start talking and to continue talking until all of the questions are answered. This technique is used to avoid short answers from the

---

*Verwoerdt, A.: Communication with the fatally ill, Springfield, Ill. 1966, Charles C Thomas, Publisher.

patient. When it works, it is great; however, the effectiveness of the multiple question technique is low. More often, the multiple question approach leads to confusion on the part of the patient. The patient may feel rushed, put down, confused, or pushed. If any of these feelings are present, the patient is unlikely to be meaningfully productive with needed information.

Silence that occurs without clear direction or meaning to the patient has been referred to as stumped silence. In stumped silence uncertainty prevails. It appears that you, the interviewer, are confused, lost, and not sure what to do next. The patient is also lost and does not know what is expected of him/her. The situation is awkward for both of you. It is better to be more specific and say, "I'm not sure that I understand," rather than stay silent and let the patient wonder what is going on. It also helps you to control your own feelings and reactions so that you can identify and verbalize them. We can always adjust better to the known than to the unknown. The patient will be much more likely to adjust to the uncertainty if it can be talked about, rather than if he/she is left with all kinds of suspicions and unsure thoughts.

Another interviewing trap is the hasty reassurance. There is almost nothing more effective for closing a topic to discussion than jumping in with, "I'm sure it will be all right." Hasty reassurance always closes the topic to discussion. When gathering data, this is the last thing you want to happen. When you need more data, reassurance will block your attempts. It is much more reassuring to be able to talk about a difficult problem than it is to have someone offer you a reassuring comment.

When the process of the data gathering produces defensiveness in the patient or in the interviewer, the effectiveness of the interview suffers. Defensiveness is usually a by-product of criticism, which is experienced as embarrassment, discomfort, shame, or rejection. Remember, it is not your job to be a *judge*. It is your job to *understand* and help the patient attain his/her goals for him/herself, not goals that you impose on the patient. It is your job to let the patient be aware of alternate goals, but it is the patient's job to select which goal he/she wishes to move toward.

A common trap in informing a patient about a procedure, a treatment, or how to take medications is to assume that the patient understands what you said in the same way you understood it when you explained it. If the patient does not understand it in the same way, the fault may not be in an inadequate explanation, but in not checking out how the communication was received and understood. Occasionally, the meaning of your words is quite different from the patient's understanding of them. The rule is to constantly check out what is being heard and understood. Occasionally, nonverbal clues will alert you that the patient must have heard something that you did not intend.

Closely allied to the patient's understanding of your words is the trap of using jargon. When professional jargon is used, the patient may feel put down, misunderstand what you say, and be very confused. We are so accustomed to jargon that we are not aware of its use until we notice a patient's confusion. This confusion will sometimes be made evident by a question indicating that the patient understands far less than we realized or by a patient just failing to follow our treatment program. When the patient fails to follow our plans for treatment, our first reaction often is that the patient is just being difficult. It is more productive to explore his/her misunderstandings. Excessive jargon contributes to misunderstandings.

8 Closing the interview

In the dental office there are two closings that take place during a visit. The first is after the initial gathering of data, at which time the actual dental procedure begins. The second is at the end of the visit.

Since the "message is in the receiver," it is important at the beginning of the dental procedure to review with the patient your understanding of what he/she has told you. If you have not already reviewed with the patient what you have heard as you proceeded during the interview and data gathering, it is wise to review with summary statements what you have heard the patient say. For example, the following summary will clarify any misunderstandings:

Well, let me review how I understand what you have told me. You first noticed the pain in your tooth when you drank ice water about 4 days ago. Since that time your tooth has continued to be sensitive to hot and cold drinks and food. You have not had any dental trouble or visits for 4 years. Your last dentist was in another city, and he put in three fillings 4 years ago. Is this information correct as you recall it?

Following this summary of the information, the patient is given an opportunity to correct any misunderstandings that you have.

One additional step is necessary before you begin the dental procedure: you need to review your contract with the patient so that both of you are clear as to what is going to take place next. You might state this in the following manner:

Now I want to check your teeth and gums, and then we will most likely need to x-ray your teeth. Once that is completed and a diagnosis is established, we can discuss what I recommend that we do to correct your difficulties. Any questions before we proceed?

The second closing, at the end of the patient's visit, is made up of three elements: (1) the final statement, (2) the prescription for action, and (3) the physical parting.

The *final statement* is a succinct survey of what you have learned and done during the visit. It is a summary of where you and the patient are in the progress of treatment. It should contain no new information but should review in a positive manner the interaction with the patient. Above all, it should contain no critical comments or any comments that belittle any of your efforts. The final statement should contain optimism that is appropriate to the patient's condition.

The *prescription for action* gives the patient a constructive plan. There is a distinction between a prescription for action and the giving of advice. A prescription for action should be based on dental knowledge. Advice is often based on little more than a hunch or personal feeling and can be given by anyone. The prescription for action is derived from the professional's expertise; it is not available from just anyone.

The prescription for action should contain your specific instructions and encourage the patient to accept responsibility for his/her share of the dental treatment. Instructions for the care, use, cleaning, and possible discomforts from the dental treatment are contained in the prescription for action.

The *physical parting* can be most awkward when another patient is waiting. The patient leaving may want or need 1 more minute, since he/she finally has his/her mouth empty of dental hardware and has had 15 or so minutes to think of all he/she wanted to say and could not. On the other hand, you feel the pressure to see the next patient. You can ease this awkwardness in several ways. Plan to have 1 or 2 minutes available for the patient to talk after his/her mouth is empty. Schedule your work so that you are not caught with too little time. Pay full attention to the patient. One minute of your undivided attention will satisfy the patient more than 5 minutes of your divided attention.

It is important that you be in charge of the door to the work area. You open the door and escort the patient out of the room to the receptionist-bookkeeper, who handles the necessary billing and scheduling for the next visit.

Question: During your first visit with a patient who has come in as a result of a decayed tooth that had become sensitive, you have checked his teeth, taken x-ray films, prepared the cavity, taken an impression, and applied a temporary filling. The visit is over. You plan to see the patient again in 3 days. Describe your procedure for terminating the visit.

Answer: *Final statement:*
We're all done for this visit. This is a temporary filling. I do not expect it to give you any trouble. If you do have any trouble, just give me a call. I will need to see you in 3 or 4 days, and at that time I will remove this temporary filling and put in the permanent inlay.
Prescription for action:
You can eat normally with this filling. Brush your teeth as you always do; just avoid picking and flossing the area of the filling. Do you have any questions?
Physical parting (after the patient's questions are answered):
Okay, now let me show you to the receptionist so that you can schedule another appointment.

This type of closing contains all of the essential elements. It is concise and leaves the patient feeling that there has been a closure to the session. The session is put into perspective. The essential treatment plan is restated so that the patient knows what he is expected to do and not to do. It also gives the patient an opportunity to ask questions and clarify directions.

The feelings common at the parting of people are sadness, anger, and appreciation. The following rhyme sums up the point: "When we part, we may be *sad, mad,* and *glad,* but that ain't *bad.*" Occasionally an additional feeling of fear or fright is present. The ultimate parting is by death. All of these feelings can be found in the surviving friends and relatives. Obviously, in comparison with a death these feelings are present in very minuscule amounts when a patient is leaving a dental appointment. The feelings may be present in all concerned, the dentist, the patient, the assistant, the receptionist, and so on. The amount of the feelings present depends on the amount of personal closeness or emotional involvement.

As we leave this chapter, we may recognize one or more of these feelings in ourselves. We have some feelings as we complete the writing of this topic.

SECTION III PATIENT BEHAVIORS

9 The cooperative patient

One of the essentials that leads to having a satisfied patient is having the patient's cooperation during the course of the dental care. The cooperative patient is one who follows directions, holds his/her mouth open sufficiently to get the work done, takes medications that are prescribed in the manner prescribed, comes for appointments, takes appropriate care of his/her dental work and teeth, and so on. This type of patient cooperates with the dentist in his/her dental care or management.

Some of the factors that lead to patient-dentist cooperation are mutual trust, the patient's feeling that the dentist cared, the patient's belief in the dentist (that the dentist is honest, good, competent, and concerned), mutual respect, a mutual feeling of being able to communicate and be understood, and both persons being in a "you count" position.

This chapter focuses on trust.

TRUST

What is the source of trust in one individual for another? Why do some people trust when others in the same situation do not trust? Is a sense of personal security within the individual important to the establishment of trust?

Question: When an individual does not trust another, there are many indicators that the trust does not exist. What are some of these indicators?

Answer: Hesitant speech
Guarded postures
Anxiety
Strong need to please
Inability to say no
Testing behavior to see if the other person can be trusted
Broken appointments
False airs, phoniness
A reaction within yourself of feeling uneasy in the presence of the other person

Once you are aware of another person's lack of trust, how do you go about understanding it? To understand lack of trust, perhaps it is necessary to first understand trust.

Trust develops from very personal experiences that are unique for each individual. Once trust in a specific relationship develops, it can then be generalized to other individuals and to institutions.

Trust may be viewed as developing from a series of behavior predictions made by one individual about another that are in harmony with what the other individual says he/she will do or be and then actually does or is. This predictive accuracy must be consistent over a number of experiences for an individual to develop trust in a second individual.

In the professional office the development of, or lack of, trust usually depends on the actuality of what the professional says will or will not happen. If you say, "This will not hurt," whether it does or does not hurt makes a difference in the development of the patient's trust. If you say, "I will see you next Tuesday at 11:00," whether you see that patient at 11:00 or 11:25 makes a difference. Each of these situations leads to the ability of the patient to accurately predict your behavior and learn that what you say can (or cannot) be trusted.

How can a patient trust a dental professional who says, "This won't hurt," and then it does? Or a professional who says, "I will see you at 11:00" and then doesn't see the patient until 11:25? What should the patient do when the dentist says, "Take these tablets at noon each day for 10 days." Should the patient take them at 1:00 for 13 days? How can the patient trust what the dental professional says when what he/she tells the patient is not true as the patient experiences it?

Once a person can trust one other person (one dentist) then that person is more likely to transfer or generalize this trust to other persons (other dentists) and will continue to trust until he/she finds a person (a dentist) that he/she cannot trust. For most of us this development of trust, or lack of it, started before we were able to remember specific events. It started with our relationship with our parenting persons in our first year of life and continues to be tested and revised every day.

From trusting specific family members, friends, and associates, we develop a generalized trust in others, such as the bus driver, the airline pilot, the other driver on the street, the banker, and the government. As the list expands, we realize that the trust in many of these individuals is blind in the sense that we will never know these people as individuals or have any personal experience with them. We trust them, however, because we have a general feeling of trust in others.

In some individuals, a lack of trust in others leads them to alter their life so as to avoid being placed in situations where they are forced to be dependent on others. Some persons' refusal to fly is based on this lack of trust in mechanics, pilots, ground controllers, electronics, machines, and so on. For a moment, consider what life would be like if you were unable to trust those around you— how you would always have to be in control of everything, leaving nothing to others, never being dependent, always being alert, never sleeping for fear that somebody might harm you. Can you get a feeling of the magnitude of the burden carried by a person who has trouble trusting others?

Do not take the patient's difficulty in trusting you lightly. It is a serious problem for the patient and for you. Respect the magnitude of this problem. Be aware that you must do what you say you will do and that you must make accurate statements about what you expect the patient to feel or not feel as you work on him/her. Keep your appointments at the time you say; if you are delayed, get a message to the patient that you expect to see him/her in a certain number of minutes and ask whether he/she prefers to wait or be rescheduled. Your failure to carry out the contract of seeing the patient at the appointed time cancels the contract, and a new contract needs to be negotiated. Once you fail to keep the appointed time, the patient is free to leave and seek another appointment time. The patient may, out of courtesy to you, wait until you are ready to see him. The opposite holds true also; out of courtesy to the patient, you may wait for him/her when he/she is delayed.

Trust between two persons is effected by the observations of the individuals involved. Because "believing is seeing," when a person generally trusts others, he/she will "see" trust in what you do and say. Likewise, when a person generally distrusts others, he will "see" distrust in what you do and say. You may have to confront such a person who distrusts with the fact that he/she did not believe or trust you about a certain matter but in fact he/she could have done so because you did what you said you would do. Thus, it may take a very active, aggressive assault on the distrust to establish a trusting relationship.

Examples of trust

Perhaps one of the first signs of lack of trust is the failure of a patient to carry out his/her part of the treatment. An example is when a patient obviously has not taken proper care of his/her teeth after being instructed in how to care for them during a previous visit.

Question: A patient has not brushed his teeth properly after having had instruction. What would you say to him to correct this situation?

Answer: You need to first establish a common understanding. The patient does not know that you think he has not followed your directions. You do not know when, how, or how often the patient has brushed his teeth. What you do know is that the result that you wanted has not occurred. Thus, a supportive confrontation or sharing of information and beliefs is needed to establish what exactly has taken place since you last saw the patient.

Question: Which of the following would you say to the patient:
A. How have you been caring for your teeth since I last saw you?
B. Something is not going as it should; your teeth seem to be much worse, as though you have not been taking care of them. How are you caring for them?
C. How are you brushing your teeth?
D. How often are you brushing your teeth?
E. It looks as though you have been having trouble caring for your teeth.
F. It looks as though you have been having trouble caring for your teeth. Does that agree with what you feel?
G. Gee! These teeth are awful! Can't you brush them the way I told you? There is no point in my doing any more work on them until you take care of them.

Answer: A, B, E, and F support the patient and open the topic for the patient to tell you what he has experienced. All except A let the patient know what you are thinking and give the patient some idea of why you are asking the questions and seeking the information.

C and *D* ask for very specific information, implying that you already know exactly what is the trouble.

G will drive the patient away unless you have a very secure, trusting relationship with him.

Question: A patient presents a very guarded posture while you are working on a filling. Assuming that the patient is able to talk to you (no dams in place), which of the following would you choose to say:

A. Now, just relax.

B. There is nothing to be afraid of.

C. You seem to have become tense. Are you aware of that?

D. You seem to be uncomfortable. Am I reading you correctly?

E. You seem to be uncomfortable. Is there something we can do to make you more comfortable?

F. What are you thinking that is making you tense and defensive or scared?

Answer: *C*, *D*, and *E* tell the patient what you have noticed and ask for verification of what is going on inside. *C* focuses on the patient's awareness of internal feelings. *D* does much the same thing but focuses on whether there is agreement between each of your understandings of what the patient is feeling. *E* focuses on treating the situation and bypasses any idea that your observations may be a misunderstanding of the patient's feelings.

A and *B* are examples of the magic of words. Say it and it will be so. The words heal. If you see your role as that of a witch doctor, select and use these responses. In practice you cannot change how another human being feels by just commanding or telling this person how he/she should feel.

F is the ideal response with a psychologically sophisticated patient. This response strikes at the heart of the problem and will lead to a correction of the tension if the patient is able to understand and control thoughts and resultant feelings. Do not use this response with a patient who has not had psychologic training, in either growth experiences, personal therapy, or sensitivity–encounter group experiences.

The last response *(F)* of the above alludes to the process of tension and the resultant defensiveness in the dental chair as we understand it. While the work is going on, the patient is thinking something. When the patient changes in his/her degree of comfort or relaxation, most likely (if you haven't done anything specific, such as cause strong pain or change procedures) the patient has had some sort of frightening thought. Focusing on this thought will bring out old fears of the patient that are associated with the thought. Focusing the patient's thoughts on something else will change the patient's feelings and thus the patient's degree of comfort.

10 Nonverbal communication

Nonverbal communication may be defined as *all channels of communication* between two humans other than the literal meaning of the words being spoken.

Question: Which of the following could be considered nonverbal communication:
A. Voice inflection, tone, and volume
B. Gesture and posture
C. Touch
D. Dress and grooming
E. Physical distance
F. Facial expression
G. Skin color (pale, blushing, and so on)
H. Care of teeth

Answer: All of the above communicate something about the person non-verbally. These nonverbal communications place the verbal communication into a context, give the words additional meaning, and on occasion belie the true meaning (which may be the opposite of the verbal words) of what the speaker honestly feels or thinks. One common example is when a person makes a positive statement and simultaneously is shaking his/her head no. Which do you believe? The verbal or the nonverbal communication? Do actions really speak louder than words?

Those who study communication have several beliefs that seem to be justified:
1. A communication has little meaning out of context. One must know the sender, the context, and the intended receiver to know the full meaning of a communication.
2. A student in a class must listen to the same lecturer for an average of 8 hours before the student can fully understand the lecturer. The greater the difference in cultural and ethnic backgrounds, the more hours are required to reach full understanding.
3. The most significant aspect of a message is that part of the message assimilated by the receiver.

69

What are the implications of these beliefs on the practices of the dental staff?

Question: Applying the first belief, that the context of a message gives the message meaning, consider the statement "My tooth hurts." What does this statement mean in each of the following circumstances:

A. A seventh-grade student speaking to his mother at 8 AM on a school morning on the day of a test for which preparation has been incomplete.

B. A 35-year-old executive speaking to a dentist during an emergency appointment. The executive has not been in a dental office in 6 years and has had no previous dental complaints. She got word yesterday that her husband was suing for divorce.

C. A 73-year-old retired college professor speaking to his dentist 2 weeks after having a new partial prosthesis.

Answer: Each of these statements might be translated as follows (other translations may be equally valid):

A. Mother, do I have to go to school today? *or* Will you let me stay home?

B. I need someone to show some interest in me.

C. I believe that this denture needs some adjusting.

The second belief, about understanding a lecturer, may be more obvious yet more abstract and difficult to document. Each patient is unique in his/her use of language to describe symptoms. Some patients describe in great detail a very precise awareness of sensation, and others barely indicate that they have an uncomfortable sensation. Before we can understand the patient's meaning of the words he/she uses, we must have some acquaintance with the person and his/her ethnic and cultural background.

Question: What would it mean to a patient if you said, "Your next appointment will be at 10 AM on the sixth of next month."

Answer: The statement would mean different things to different people, depending on their cultural expectations.* Some patients might interpret this statement to mean that they should arrive at the dental office before noon on the sixth. Others would be likely to arrive at 9:45 on the sixth. Still others might interpret the statement to mean that they should come if any discomfort persists. If there is no discomfort, there is no obligation to come.

The third belief, that the most significant aspect of a message is that part of the message assimilated by the receiver, is an important element in the treatment of a patient.

Question: What would it mean to a patient if you said, "Take one of these pills when the pain becomes severe."

---

*Saunders, L.: Cultural difference and medical care, New York, 1954, Russel Sage Foundation.

Answer: Possible meanings to the patient might be:

The dentist wants me to suffer some.

The pills are powerful, so don't take very many of them.

Never take two pills at one time.

Don't try to relieve the pain in any other way.

The pills will relieve any kind of pain.

The pills only work on severe pains.

Don't take the pills unless you just have to.

Take only these pills, no others, for pain.

The pain is important; tend to it carefully.

The difference between what we mean to say and what we say (and how it is interpreted) is often surprising. If you have had little experience with word meanings or interpretations, do the following exercise with another person and then discuss what each of you have learned. The rules of the exercise are:

1. Person *A* makes a statement to person *B*. The statement can be about anything and should have some significance to *A*. For example, "I would like to know you better."
2. *B* asks questions of *A* as follows: "By that, do you mean. . . ?"
3. *A* can answer *only* by saying yes or no.
4. *B* must obtain three yes answers from *A*.

This exercise is referred to as a "make meaning exercise" and has been most productive of learning when used with dental, dental hygiene, and medical students.

If you were *B* in the exercise, you may have noted that you used some nonverbal clues to guide you to an understanding of the meaning of the message. The payoff of this exercise (and the understanding of the principles involved) occurs when you are giving directions to patients. Remembering that the "message is in the receiver" should encourage you to inquire of the patient what the patient heard you say and what that means to the patient. In checking out what the patient heard, you may frequently learn that the patient was more tuned in to nonverbal messages from you than to the words that you were using.

VALUE OF READING NONVERBALS

There are many possible ways that reading the patient's nonverbal messages will help you in the dental office:

1. You will have a more accurate understanding of what the patient means when he/she is talking.
2. Nonverbals give instantaneous information. You don't have to wait for the end of a statement to learn the speaker's meaning.
3. If your reading of the nonverbals tells you whether the patient is sad, mad, glad, scared, or anxious, your response to the patient can be appropriate to the patient's feelings state (affect). For example, your response to a sad person would be quite different from your response to an angry person. If you do not read the nonverbals, you may not be aware of the affect of the patient.
4. The patient's instantaneous reaction to your last action or response may only be available to you through the reading of nonverbal clues. As an ongoing process without constant nonverbal feedback, the interaction may enter into mutual monologues, with each of you expressing yourself as though the other person were not present.

5. When you give the patient such complete attention that you read his/her nonverbals, the patient is flattered, feels positively toward you, and feels that he/she has finally found someone who can understand. When such positive rapport exists, malpractice suits are extremely rare, faithful patients are the rule, enjoyment in the dental practice is common, and night calls to clarify misunderstanding are rare.
6. The patient is impressed when he/she is the center of your attention. Your concern, care, and interest for the patient are apparent. Who can fail to want to cooperate when this kind of attention is being given?
7. A patient appreciates your concern for him/her as a human being, a person, rather than as a tooth, a body with teeth in it, a dental rarity, or an oral cavity.
8. The information that you obtain simultaneously through more than one channel of communication is more reliable than information from a single channel. The words alone may mislead, just as nonverbal clues used alone may mislead. When touch, sounds, words, body language, gestures, and facial expressions are all considered together, the true meaning of a communication is rarely missed. Each clue either substantiates your impression from the previous clue or contradicts the previous clue.
9. Since the patient finds it difficult to talk when your hand and tools are in his/her mouth, nonverbal channels of communication are at times all that is available from him/her.

FRAMEWORK FOR READING NONVERBALS

It is helpful to have a framework within which meaning can be given to nonverbal clues. One effective method of organizing nonverbal information is to consider whether a person is being open or closed to a new idea or thought when he/she expresses the nonverbal. Another method is to organize the information according to the affect (feeling) of the individual when he/she expresses a certain nonverbal.

Open versus closed

A person is open to a new idea or thought when he/she has some comfort and security with the situation, does not feel too threatened or anxious, and has the energy necessary to consider something new. A person who is too exhausted, in too much pain, too scared, too angry, or too sad will not be open to a new idea or thought. Frequently these internal states are reflected by body posture.

Question: Determine whether the body posture in each of the following drawings suggests that the person is open or closed to a new idea or thought.

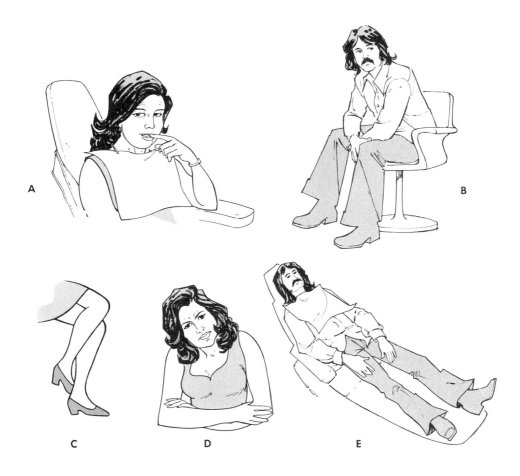

Answer: *A, B,* and *E* are considered by most observers to be the postures that signal openness to a new idea or thought. The remaining postures are considered closed. Persons in these postures are much less frequently open to a new idea.

In the dental office a patient's open or closed posture may be especially important when you are ready to give the patient instructions concerning his/her treatment.

Question: If you are ready to give instructions and find that the patient is in a closed posture, what do you do?

Answer: Determine what the patient is thinking about, what is on his/her mind, and deal with the problem at hand until the patient shifts to a more open posture. Then give your instructions. If the patient does not move to a more open posture, ask the patient if he/she is ready for the instructions about his/her further treatment.

Question: What posture do you want the patient to be in when you give instructions concerning the treatment? Should the patient be lying down, sitting up, or standing? Should the patient be above your eye level, at your eye level, or below your eye level?

Answer: Generally, you want to talk to the rational, computer part of the patient when you give him/her directions.

If you have the patient lying down in the dental chair, he/she tends to be in a dependent, childlike ego state. If you give directions to this part of the patient, he/she may react to the directions in much the same way that a child would.

At the other extreme, if you have the patient standing over you, above you, or in a more controlling position, he/she tends to be in a dominant, parentlike ego state. The patient may then react to your directions much as a parent would to directions given by a child.

Thus, directions will have a greater chance of being carried out in a rational manner if they are given to the patient when he/she is seated at a height equal to yours. When the patient is at an equal height, in an upright position, he/she tends to be in the adult or computer ego state and will tend to react in a more rational manner.*

Affectual states

Your reactions to the patient will differ depending on both the mood or affect of the patient and your own mood or affect at the time. Therefore, it is useful to have some paradigm by which moods or affects can be identified. Plutchik has developed one useful paradigm.† According to Plutchik, the primary affectual states are the unpleasurable states of sadness, anxiety, anger, and disgust, the state of comfort, and the pleasurable states of happiness, joy, and excitement.

Most observers, with no training, have little difficulty reading the pleasurable affectual states of happiness, joy, and excitement. Difficulty more frequently occurs in reading the unpleasurable affectual states of sadness, anxiety, anger, and disgust and in thereby reacting appropriately to the situation. For example, the reaction to a sad person would be quite different from the reaction to a person who is angry.

Anxiety. Anxiety is a common affectual state. It arises from a real or imagined threat. The threat may be real, that is, observed by others to exist, or it may be imagined, that is, believed by the individual but unable to be observed by others. The threat may be the possibility of loss of a tooth, job, health, life, or love. Real threats include events such as an automobile coming toward you, a hand holding pliers and coming toward your mouth, or a barking dog lunging toward you. Imagined threats may include unconfirmed beliefs such as your boss mistrusting you, your spouse loving another person, or you having a dreaded disease.

---

*See James, M., and Jongeward, D.: Born to win, Reading, Mass., 1971, Addison-Wesley Publishing Co., Inc., for a discussion of ego states.

†Plutchik, R.: The emotions: facts, theories, and a new model, New York, 1962, Random House, Inc.

Question: Which of the following words would the anxious person use to describe him/herself? "I am . . . "
A. Shy
B. Annoyed
C. Sad
D. Tired
E. Nervous
F. Anxious
G. Apprehensive

Answer: A, E, F, and G are words frequently used by the anxious person.

Question: How would the anxious person complete the following sentence? "I feel like . . . "
A. Hitting
B. Running
C. Shaking
D. Going away
E. Vomiting
F. Laughing
G. Hiding

Answer: B, C, E, and G are feelings frequently expressed by the anxious person.

Question: Select the drawing in each of the following pairs that best portrays anxiety.

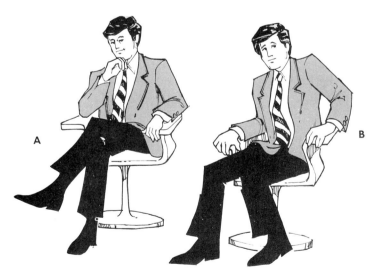

A   B

Continued.

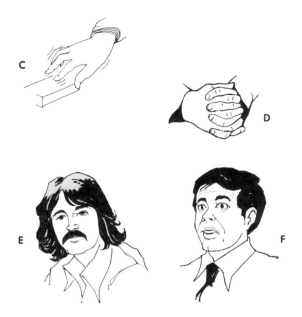

Answer: *B, C,* and *F* best portray anxiety. The anxious facial expression may include a raised forehead, raised eyebrows, eyelids open wide to see where the danger is coming from, dilated pupils, a round, open mouth, trembling lips, and a licking of the lips. In addition, the face may be white with cold sweat. The anxious person's bodily expressions may include a fixed head, as though he/she were pulling away, gestures of guarding him/herself, trembling, a posture of being ready for flight, and trivial hand occupation.

Question: What is the respiration like in the anxious person? Describe the rate and depth of respiration, and going back to physiology, the efficiency of this type of breathing.

Answer: The anxious person breathes more rapidly than normal. The depth of respiration is very shallow. When the rapid rate is combined with the shallow excursion, little air is moved and very little oxygen is exchanged in the alveoli. Thus, the efficiency is decreased, and a mild anoxia exists. Some authorities believe that if the amount of oxygen (oxygen tension) in the blood is increased in a person who is anxious, the person will feel less anxious and more comfortable.

Question: According to the last answer, what would you do to enable an anxious person to feel less anxious and more comfortable?

Answer: You would encourage the person to breathe more slowly and with deeper respirations. One technique is to have the person count to four during each of the following: inspiration, holding breath in, expiration, and holding breath out. The person should then repeat the cycle until he/she is more comfortable.

Question: Which one of the following drawings portrays the gait of the anxious person?

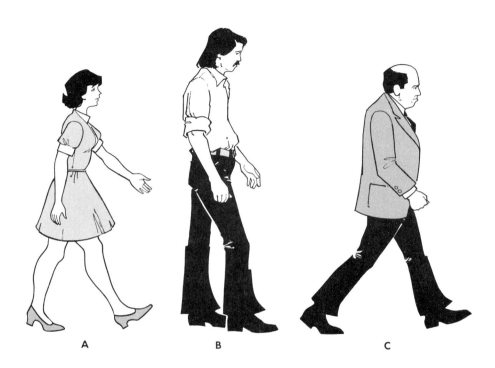

A　　　　　　　　B　　　　　　　　C

Answer: *A* depicts the gait of the anxious person. It is careful and cautious, with head erect, eyes searching for danger, and weight centered between the feet; the body is erect, and the stride is usually lengthened. The walk of the anxious person shows the energy that is in check but available.

Anger. Anger is the normal response to frustration. When progress toward a goal is impeded, a person is frustrated in moving toward his/her goal, and the resulting physiologic changes and behavior are described as aggression or anger. Anger resulting from a stimulus that is nonobstructive, that does not interfere in the reaching of goals, is considered neurotic.

Question: Which of the following drawings portray the angry person?

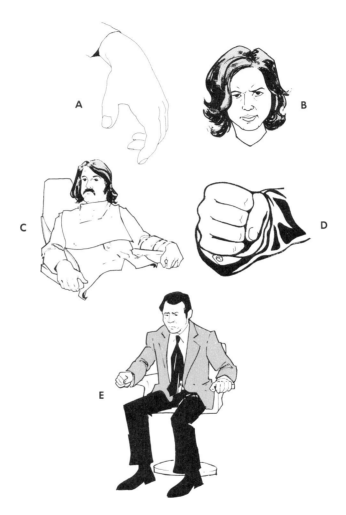

Answer: *B, D,* and *E* are examples of nonverbal expressions of anger. Note that the angry face has a frowning forehead with knit eyebrows; the eyelids are narrowed, and the eyes are looking straight at the barricade that impedes the progress. The mouth is open in an elliptical, tense grin; the teeth are clinched, and the lips are compressed and retracted. The neck veins are prominent (distended), the face is red, the masseter muscles are tight and the nostrils are widened. The head is tilted forward with the chin protruding.

Question: Which of the following words would the angry person use to describe him/herself? "I am . . . "
A. Fearful
B. Annoyed
C. Dejected
D. In a rage
E. Disinterested
F. Mad
G. Bad
H. Irritated
I. Angry

Answer: *B, D, E, F, G, H,* and *I* are words frequently used by the person who is angry.

Question: How would the angry person complete the following sentence? "I feel like . . . "
A. Hiding
B. Giving up
C. Hitting
D. Shouting
E. Crying
F. Slamming the door
G. Killing
H. Running

Answer: *C, D, F,* and *G* are feelings frequently expressed by the angry person.

Question: How would you describe the gait of the angry person?

Answer: The gait of the angry person may be portrayed by the following drawing.

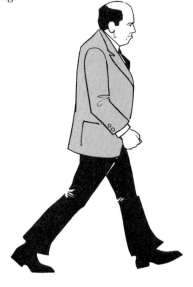

In the gait of the angry person the weight is forward, the head is forward and up so that the eyes are looking straight ahead, the hands are in the form of a fist, and the arms are rigid. This person is ready to fight with the obstacle in his/her way.

Question: Describe the respiration and speech of the angry person.

Answer: The respiration is forceful, with speech occurring during the middle of expiration. The speech comes in staccato bursts or outbursts and may be forceful, loud, and precise.

Grief or sorrow. Grief or sorrow is the feeling that is the normal response to loss. The loss may be that of a loved one, friend, object, part of oneself (such as a tooth), pet, or position. The loss of respect, freedom, or faith may also be considered significant losses.

Question: Which of the following words would a person use to describe him/herself when grieving or sorrowful? "I am . . . "
A. Dejected
B. Irritated
C. Anxious
D. Pensive
E. Depressed
F. Tired
G. Gloomy
H. Sad

Answer: *A, D, E, G,* and *H* are the words used by the person who is experiencing grief or sorrow.

Question: How would such a person complete the following sentence? "I feel like . . . "
A. Giving up
B. Running away
C. Hitting
D. Crying
E. Falling apart
F. Going away
G. Empty
H. Dying

Answer: *A, D, F, G,* and *H* are feelings frequently expressed by the person who has experienced a loss. Remember, running away is an expression of the anxious person. The sad person does not have the energy available that the anxious or angry person has.

Question: How might you help a person who has just suffered a loss to cope with the loss more effectively?

Answer: Since this person does not have much energy available, you should do anything that you can to help the person get in touch with his/her energy. First, allow the person to grieve, to cry, and to be sad, but then help the person to return to activities that are normal for him/her. This will generate interest and energy to live.

Question: Which of the following drawings portray the person who is grieving?

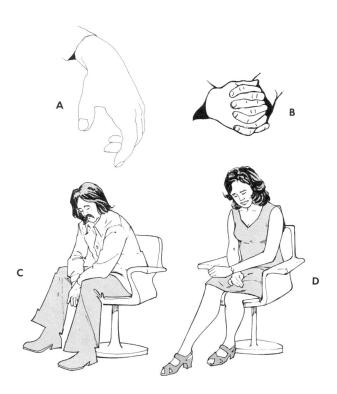

Answer: *A, C,* and *D* depict expressions of sorrow. The sad, grieving person has the forehead flat and the eyes half closed and downcast; the eyes may be red with tears; the mouth is in the form of an inverted crescent; the face is pale and lengthened, and the muscles are flaccid. It is as though there were no nervous impulses to the muscles of the face and they were being pulled by gravity.

Question: Describe the speech and respiration of the grieving person.

Answer: The respirations are slow, sighing, and shallow. The speech is soft, slow, and weeping and occurs at the end of expiration. Air is exhaled in a sigh, and then the person speaks.

Question: Describe the posture and gait of the grieving person.

Answer: The posture of the sad, grieving person may be described as the body hanging by the ligaments. It is as though there were no muscle tone or muscular help in holding the body erect. The head is hanging. The limbs are limp, and there are few gestures except for some hand wringing. The gait is slouched, weight is back on the feet, and steps tend to be short and slow. Abdominal muscles sag, and the abdomen is protuberant. Arms are relaxed. It is as though the person were saying to the world: "Come hit me, for I must be bad and deserve to be punished. I am defenseless and will [can] *not* put up a fight." Another reading of this posture may be "I am helpless; come take care of me."

The following drawing depicts the gait of the sad person.

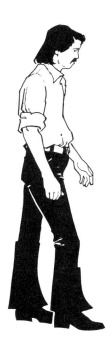

Disgust. Disgust is the physiologic response to a noxious situation or stimuli. The situation or stimulus is one to which the person can *not* be comfortable.

Question: Which of the following words would the disgusted person use to describe him/herself? "I am . . . "
A. Bored
B. Nauseated
C. Annoyed
D. Dejected
E. Tired
F. Loathing
G. Disinterested

Answer: *A, B, E,* and *F* are words frequently used by the disgusted person.

Question: How would the disgusted person complete the following sentence: "I feel like . . ."
A. Vomiting
B. Crying
C. Hiding
D. Bashing in a wall
E. Turning away
F. Running

Answer: *A*, *C*, and *E* are feelings frequently expressed by the disgusted person.

Question: Which of the following drawings portray the digusted person?

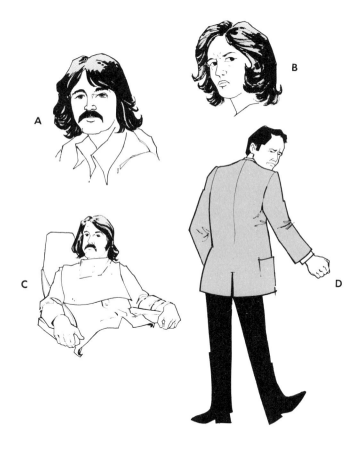

Answer: *B* and *D* depict nonverbal expressions of disgust. The face of the disgusted person has some frowning of the forehead; the eyes squint occasionally and turn away. The mouth may show a sneer or the early signs of imminent vomiting. The head is generally turned away from the object or person causing the disgust. The posture of the disgusted person is primarily that of turning or pushing away, with a hand moving to the abdomen or mouth as if catching an uncomfortable part of the body.

Question: Describe the speech and respiration of the disgusted person.

Answer: The speech is snorting or snearing. The respiration is halting; there is a tendency toward hesitation.

Question: When might you expect to observe a reaction of disgust in the dental patient?

Answer: Obviously, the reaction will occur following the presentation of something to the patient. It might be an instrument, a mouthwash, a plastic to make an impression, or a new partial denture; it might be a treatment plan or a recommendation for care. In these situations it may be very important to be alert to such a reaction by the patient.

Question: You have just presented the treatment plan to a patient and have observed a reaction that you interpret to be one of disgust. How would you proceed?

Answer: There are several ways to proceed. One way might be to comment on the patient's reaction. When you make this type of confrontation, you should use a congruent statement, one in which you take full responsibility for your observation of disgust, and one in which you allow the patient to deal with this reaction. You should not be critical of the reaction; the patient has every right to dislike your plan. The following responses fill these requirements:

I detect some discomfort on your part to this treatment plan.
I sense that you are not pleased with this treatment plan.

SECTION IV PRACTICE INTERVIEWS AND COMMUNICATION SIMULATIONS

A delayed office schedule

Mr. King is a business executive in his early forties. He has a top-level position in a very large firm and seems used to making important decisions quickly. He has been kept waiting about 15 minutes past his appointment time. He is now seated with the receptionist.

Receptionist: I'm awfully sorry to have kept you waiting. Sometimes things just seem to get out of hand.

Question: What does this statement by the receptionist really say?

Answer: I know that I've kept you waiting. Don't be angry with me. I'm helpless; I'm not responsible. You're a *big* person, and I'm a little receptionist. You count and I don't count.

King: I know. I'm always having trouble with my secretaries, too.

Translation: You're as bad as my secretaries, who are also incompetent.

Receptionist: (Looking up quickly and then returning her gaze back to the chart on her desk.) Well, what I meant was that we can't always predict things that happen in the office, things with patients, you know.

Translation: You know, patients are just as bad. They don't keep to a schedule, either. Sometimes they're late or take up more time than they should.

King: I explained when I made the appointment that I keep a tight schedule. I hope the doctor is able to work within it.

Translation: I really mean work with *me*—I'm as important as the dentist.

Receptionist: Oh, we try very hard to be efficient. We're very organized around here.

Translation: We know we're not very efficient, but we play the game that we're *trying* to be efficient. We mask the lack of efficiency with a lot of motion and apologies.

Comment: This interview has gotten off to an unfortunate start and might reasonably be expected to proceed in the following manner.

Receptionist: Well, I see from your record that everything is more or less okay. You do have a history of some allergies and you've had an operation for an ulcer—is that right?

King: Yes.

Receptionist: Oh! I believe that the doctor is ready for you. I suppose we can get more about that later on. Please come this way.

Comment: Intimidated by the dentist's lateness and perhaps by the presence of this VIP, the receptionist, in her anxiety to atone for perceived failure, may really be neglecting some important areas of information. Thus, this interview is essentially nonproductive. The receptionist is unduly defensive and either wishes the patient to think better of her or is seeking to protect her boss's reputation as an efficient manager. If the delay was indeed unavoidable, an appropriate comment of apology is quite in order, but anything more simply prolongs the time before relevant information is forthcoming. A more productive statement might be the following.

Receptionist: I'm awfully sorry we couldn't get to you right on time. Something unexpected delayed our schedule, and it was too late to contact you. Now, let me get the information we need.

Ms. Arnold
conflict about personal information

Ms. Arnold is a well-groomed career woman in her mid to late thirties. This is her first visit to the dental office. She has already filled out an abbreviated medical history questionnaire. She has no predominant problems and was referred by another patient. It is not yet known why she is seeking a new dentist. She is being interviewed by the receptionist before meeting the dentist for the first time.

Receptionist: Good morning, Ms. Arnold. Thank you for being so prompt. Do you have any questions after completing the questionnaire?

Arnold: No.

Receptionist: Now, there is some information I would like to obtain from you for our records before you meet Dr. Hansen. First, do I have the correct spelling of your name?

Arnold: Yes, except my first name is spelled with an "O."

Receptionist: Good. I'm glad we caught that error. Your address is 7215 Canyon Dr., and your telephone number is 836-5927.

Arnold: Yes.

Receptionist: Your birth date was omitted. What is it?

Arnold: (Up until now the patient has responded in an expected manner.) You really don't have to know that. I'm over 21.

Question: How would you respond to this patient? Would you confront her? Would you use a facilitation, a direct question, or another type of reply? What is the issue? What is the relationship process? What is being questioned by the patient?

Answer: The patient is testing the relationship to learn something. We can only speculate on what the patient is after. Maybe she is asking: "Will you treat me as an individual?" "Does an individual's privacy count here?" "What difference does it really make how old I am?" or "If my age is that important, maybe the really important part of my life has ended?" Compare your response to the patient with the one made by the receptionist.

Receptionist: Well, we do like to have complete records for our patients, so I would like to be able to enter your birth date.

Comment: This reply ignores the patient's feelings and deals with the issues in a matter-of-fact manner. This reply says we do everything "by the book," according to the rules. It also implies that the records and procedures are more important than the people involved and their feelings. An alternate reply by the receptionist might have been, "You would rather not have your birth date on this form." If said with the connotation, "That is all right, we can deal with you as an individual; we respect your feelings and your need for keeping some information private," this reply might meet the challenge of this patient and win her over for the duration of her need for dental care. This reply also says, "I am alert to your feelings, since I just responded to them."

Arnold: Well, it's September 15, 1938.

Receptionist: And what do you do, Ms. Arnold?

Arnold: Why do you have to know that?

Question: What would you do now? How would you respond to this second irregular answer?

Answer: Instead of giving a specific answer, we will just follow one line of replies and see what happens.

Receptionist: Again, we are simply trying to obtain a complete record for our files, as we do for all our patients.

Arnold: Well, I don't see how what I do for a living has anything to do with my teeth.

Receptionist: (Getting a little frustrated or angry.) Well, how about giving us a telephone number at work?

Arnold: Really, I don't see that as being any of your business.

Receptionist: We may have to reach you to change an appointment.

Arnold: I don't want to be called at work. If I can't make it, I'll call you.

Receptionist: Well, the doctor would really like to be able to reach you, too.

Arnold: We'll see. I'll think about that.

Question: What has happened here? What was overlooked in this exchange? What is the fight all about?

Answer: The patient is a human being, a unique individual, not a depersonalized set of gums with teeth. She wants to be treated as a worthwhile person who has feelings. What was overlooked? Her feelings. The receptionist in this exchange behaved more like a computer. She did not reply to the patient's feelings and did not acknowledge them. She ignored them.

Comment: You might learn a great deal by role playing this interaction. When the patient first deviates from the expected patient role, change the receptionist's replies in a way that recognizes the patient's feelings and see what happens—how long or how short a time it takes to deal with the feelings and move to another topic with the patient being much more cooperative.

Receptionist: Okay, I see you have completed the medical history. It looks as though you're in good health. You don't have any history of heart trouble—is that correct?

Arnold: Yes.

Receptionist: Never had diabetes; no trouble with allergies to any drugs.

Comment: Generally, leading questions like these are unacceptable; but following the patient's completion of a history, they are about all that you can do.

Arnold: Yes, that's correct.

Question: With the hostile interaction that has been established between these two combatants, how reliable are these answers?

Answer: Highly unreliable (see the section in Chapter 7 on "yes" and "no" answers, p. 52).

Receptionist: Are you taking any medications now, any pills of any kind, on a regular basis?

Question: Give at least two reasons why this question is not a good one.

Answer: 1. Three questions are combined into one. Which question should the patient answer?
2. The questions are conflicting. Does the receptionist want to know if the patient is taking any pills, or does she want to know if the patient is taking any pills on a regular basis? Is a pill different from a medication? Does she mean shots or liquids by the word "medication"?

Arnold: I don't see what that has to do with dentistry.

Receptionist: I'm just inquiring as to whether you're taking any pills.

Comment: It does not sound that way to us.

Arnold: Yes, I am on the pill, but that can't possibly have anything to do with my dental condition. If any of this is necessary at all, can't I go over it with the dentist?

Receptionist:	I'm trying to save some time for the dentist, so if you can answer these questions for me before you see the dentist ...
Arnold:	Well, if they have anything to do with my health, I'll answer them directly to the dentist, if that's necessary.
Receptionist:	Have you ever had rheumatic fever?
Arnold:	No.
Receptionist:	Do you have any trouble with stopping bleeding, like when you cut yourself around the house or something?
Question:	Reword the receptionist's last question to improve it.
Answer:	Do you ever have trouble stopping a cut from bleeding? (If the answer is yes, follow up the question for additional information.)
Arnold:	Look, I said I'll talk it over with the dentist.
Receptionist:	We have to get our records complete.
Arnold:	I've gone to other dentists, and no one has ever asked me these questions; least of all, a secretary.
Receptionist:	How is it that you happened to come to our office?
Comment:	A real blow below the belt.
Arnold:	Ms. Howard, your patient, recommended Dr. Hansen. My former dentist is getting a little old, and I thought maybe he wouldn't be able to take care of me anymore.
Receptionist:	Well, I'm sure that Dr. Hansen will be able to take care of you very well. Now, just a few more questions ...
Question:	Does the dentist have any chance of establishing a successful dentist-patient relationship with this patient after her hostile interaction with the receptionist?
Answer:	It is possible, but the odds are against it. Let's follow the receptionist as she talks with the dentist.
Receptionist:	Boy, is there a winner out there! She's real hard type. Wait until you see her. Won't answer questions, wouldn't even tell me her age. Lots of luck.
Comment:	What a setup!
Dentist:	What happened out there?
Receptionist:	You'll see. We don't need patients like her around here. You'll probably want to get rid of her right away.
Comment:	Either get rid of the patient or the receptionist. Hopefully, it will not come to this choice. Remember, the patient pays the dentist, and the dentist pays the receptionist.

92

Dentist: Well, bring her in. I hope it doesn't take too much time to find out what's going on.

Question: The stage is set. The battle lines are drawn. How would you proceed if you were the dentist?

Answer: Whatever you do must fit your style. You might wish to gain a further understanding of what happened from your receptionist and help her so that she can respond differently to the next patient who reacts like this. You might give up on your receptionist in this case and plan to focus on correcting the situation with the patient so that you can salvage a cooperative patient out of the existing mess. There are several alternative ways of proceeding. We will look at three.

Dentist: My receptionist tells me there are some questions you don't wish to answer. I'm sorry, but we insist on complete records for all our patients. Most of our patients don't have any trouble answering these questions. I'm afraid I'll have to ask you where you work and if there's a telephone number where I can reach you at work. Without this information it won't be possible for us to go any further.

Comment: This response clearly draws battle lines; it establishes an "in" group of the dentist and his staff against the outsider, the patient. It also says: "We treat depersonalized robots, not real people who have feelings and differences and who are unique and require individualized reactions on our part. Our systems are more important to us than the people they serve." It is a real "I do not count; you do not count; the system does count" transaction. You may wish to function in such a system, but many persons do not.

The following is a second way of proceeding with the patient.

Dentist: I see there are some blanks on our records, Ms. Arnold. Is there something about our questions that you don't understand?

Arnold: No, it's just that some of the questions seemed too personal to come from a dentist, and certainly to come from a dentist's secretary. The other questions I just didn't think were any of her business. Also, I've gone to dentists before, and they've never asked me questions about medicines I was taking or anything like that.

Comment: The neutral tone of the dentist seeks to elicit, in the patient's own words, what the problem is. The dentist is then better able to evaluate for himself the comments of the receptionist. His replies can be directed right at the patient's concerns, and he can establish his own basis for seeking the same information.

Question: What would have been a better reply by the dentist than the question he did ask—"Is there something about our questions that you don't understand?"

Answer: This question is too narrowing, too specific. We prefer an open-ended question or facilitation. The following reply seems to us to be the best: "I see there are some blanks on our records, Ms. Arnold. I don't understand." This reply is honest and places the patient in the position to explain, from her viewpoint, what has happened. There is no judgment involved. Rather than just asking for a logical, cognitive, explanation of what has happened, this reply allows for feelings to be given as reasons. The previous question asked specifically for " . . . something about our questions you don't *understand*?" rather than " . . . something about our questions you don't *like*?" The following answers are also acceptable:

"I see there are some blanks on our records, Ms. Arnold. How come?"

"You prefer not to answer these questions?"

"These questions upset you?"

"You're not sure you can trust us with this information?"

The following is a third way of proceeding with this patient.

Dentist: Well, I'm sorry you have had some difficulties. Our receptionist was doing her job according to my instructions, and I hope she didn't offend you. Her questions were about information we have to know to provide you with our best care.

Comment: By acknowledging difficulties that the patient may have had with the receptionist and by supporting the receptionist, the dentist lets the patient know that he values his staff and does not allow his staff to act capriciously. Simultaneously, he conveys a sensitivity to the patient's needs, especially the need for an explanation. We would like to see the above statement followed by "How may we help you become comfortable with our way of running the office?" This question shows the dentist's concern and asks the patient to take responsibility for her discomfort and for the solution to her discomfort.

Dentist: Your age is important to us because it indicates how rapidly or slowly dental disease may or may not be progressing in your mouth. Obviously a cavity in the molar of a 6-year-old child is quite a different thing from a cavity of the same size in say, a middle-aged man. Also, although you may not be aware of it, many drugs that people take may interact with drugs that the dentist uses, such as Novocain. So, I hope you will be able to see that we are not prying but really want to help you. The more we know about your health, the more certain we can be that our decisions in the dental area are in your own best interests.

Arnold: Well, to tell you the truth, I never thought of it that way. I want to thank you for your explanation. I guess if your receptionist had put it to me that way, I probably wouldn't have objected so much.

Comment: At this point the interview may proceed with the specific information needed and the necessary examination of the patient.

Ms. Smith
an anxious patient

The dental assistant has been talking with the patient on the way to the operatory and is now seating Ms. Smith in the dental chair. The dentist comes in.

Assistant: And Ms. Smith wanted me to be sure to tell you that she's terrified of the dentist.

Smith: Could you lower the head thing? It's hitting me right here.

Assistant: But I told her not to worry, we were used to her type.

Smith: No, that's still too high. Just a little lower, please.

Assistant: I told her you were simply marvelous with nervous women. Isn't that right, Doctor?

Smith: Does the chair have to be tilted so far back?

Dentist: (Washing his hands with his back to the patient, so that he is talking over his shoulder.) That's right, don't worry about a thing.

Question: What does "don't worry" really say to another person?

Answer: A sentence with a *not* in it is a negative suggestion. Let us digress for a moment. Now, do not think about an elephant. Do not think about its tough skin, its big feet, its long flappy ears, and its long trunk. What are you thinking about? Oh! Really! An elephant? But we told you specifically *not* to think about an elephant. Now, we want you to think about a giraffe, with its long neck, stretching up to some tender leaves on a tree for a nourishing meal. Are you thinking about an elephant? Of course not. The point of all this is that if you want a person to worry, tell that person *not* to worry. If you do not want a person to worry, focus that person's attention on something else. The above direction, "Don't worry about a thing," can be translated as "Worry about everything."

Assistant: See, I told you. All our patients really love to come here.

Smith: Do you really need that bright light so close to my eyes?

Assistant:	This towel will help keep everything nice and neat. Now that you're comfortable, the doctor can begin his examination.
Dentist:	(Now seated on his stool and approaching the patient with a mirror and an explorer.) Now open wide, and let's see what we have here.
Comment:	This kind of impersonal, inconsiderate interaction occurs frequently. The patient verbally communicated a concern. The assistant and the dentist, preoccupied with their respective roles, duties, and busywork, acted as though they heard the patient, but their conversation did not acknowledge the presence of the patient or her concerns. Instead of "Now open wide . . . ," the dentist might have said the following.
Dentist:	Tell me how you feel about coming here.
Smith:	I don't know. It's just a lousy feeling. It's out of all proportion to anything that's ever happened to me. I just really dislike coming. It's not personal, you know; it's not you. It's just the thought of all those instruments and that drilling, that noise. I even hate the Novacain. I don't know which I hate more, the pain or the lousy feeling I get from the Novacain.
Comment:	Often, simply giving the patient a chance to ventilate feelings produces a barrage of previously inhibited statements about feelings, expectations, and immediate fears. The fact that they can be spoken, said aloud, and shared with another and nothing traumatic happens as a result, takes some of the sting out of the feelings. Some patients feel that they may be considered neurotic or crazy, if they have fears or strong feelings. The fact that the dentist or assistant can accept a patient having such feelings is reassuring to the patient. It says: "Others have these feelings; you're not abnormal. We can still help you."
Dentist:	Well, thank you for telling me how you feel. It certainly will be helpful to me in treating you. If at any time you wish to tell me anything about how the treatment is going, please do so. You can stop me by simply raising your hand. Do you have any suggestions for how you would prefer for me to proceed?
Smith:	No, not right now.
Dentist:	Maybe if I begin my oral examination now with this mirror and explorer and find out what state of health your mouth is in, I can tell you some alternative ways of being treated.
Smith:	That sounds reasonable. I hope you don't think I'm a pest or that I'm taking up too much of your time.
Comment:	This patient is in a "I don't count, you count" transaction with the dentist. Patients are often truly ambivalent about the conflict of meeting their own needs, as opposed to allowing the dentist to meet his/her needs. When the patient is given the opportunity to express his/her concerns and also has the prospect

of some control over the situation, anxiety is sufficiently reduced to allow treatment to proceed relatively routinely. Also, when given some control over the situation, the patient assumes responsibility for the continuing care of his/her dental health. If you start out with the patient in a very dependent position, flat on his/her back, you must somehow end your treatment with the patient being responsible for his/her continuing dental health. Making the patient responsible must be a part of your treatment goal and plans, or you will be drained dry from giving the milk of human kindness to each of your dependent patients.

Dentist: (With the patient sitting in an upright position so that she can assume a more responsible role.) Well, now I've finished the examination of your mouth. You were most cooperative. I know that wasn't easy for you.

Smith: I want to thank you for your patience, but the examination never really bothered me. It's the thought of those needles and that noisy drill and the feeling you get from the novocain. The feeling of being dependent and helpless is hard for me. I can't stand any of that.

Dentist: When we first began today's appointment, you seemed pretty anxious in general.

Smith: Yes, I was a little concerned at the beginning of the appointment.

Dentist: A lot of times, after people have been through the experience, they look back and see that it wasn't really so bad. Maybe you'll have that experience the next time you come, when we'll go a little further into the periodontal treatments.

Smith: You mean the gum scraping? I really don't think so, Doctor. That's a really terrible thing to do to someone.

Assistant: Well, we'll go slow, and you'll get a chance to tell us how you're doing along the way. We'll work at it together.

Dentist: That's right. We'll tell you all about it first and help you learn that a good part of what frightens you is the unknown. So far, you've done just beautifully, even though you didn't think you would.

Comment: Positive reinforcement, a sense of accomplishment, and support have been provided by the dentist and the assistant. Such positive, future-oriented, patient support actually requires very little time and is a very effective anxiety reducer. Note that the assistant is tuned in to both the patient and the dentist. The assistant's comments are appropriately timed and flow out of the same approach taken by the dentist.

It may also be noted that even though an appointment may begin very poorly, recovery can be made and a successful visit may ensue.

Mr. Arnold
a new patient to the office

Dentist:	Mr. Dean Arnold? Hi, I'm Larry McGuiness. You want to come with me?
Question:	How would you improve this opening?
Answer:	Dean Arnold? Hi, I'm Dr. Larry McGuiness. Please come this way with me.
Arnold:	Okay.
Dentist:	(After being seated.) What are you here for today?
Arnold:	Well, I've got this boil here on my gum. It's really kind of bothering me.
Dentist:	How long have you had that?
Question:	What is wrong with this reply?
Answer:	There are three things wrong with this reply:

    1. The dentist is not letting the patient tell his story.
    2. The dentist is not letting the patient take any responsibility for giving the history.
    3. The dentist is asking when something that is unknown to him began. Since he does not know what the patient is talking about, he will not be able to ask for meaningful information.

Question:	Make up a better reply to Mr. Arnold.
Answer:	Compare your replies with the following:

Bothering!
A boil?
What's it like?
What have you noticed?
How does it bother you?

Arnold:	Couple of months now . . .
Dentist:	Do you have any pain?

99

Question: What is wrong with this reply?

Answer: Again, the dentist is not letting the patient tell his story or take any responsibility for giving the history, and the question suggests that there should be pain or that the dentist expects the patient to have had pain. A suggestible patient (30% of patients are suggestible to the point of making the response unreliable) may respond to the suggestion rather than convey accurate information.

Question: Make up an alternate reply.

Answer: Compare your replies with the following:
Couple of months!
What was it like when you first noticed it?
What did you first notice?
Tell me what you remember about it.
You don't run for help for quite a while, do you?

Arnold: Well, for a while it did, but it doesn't now.

Comment: This is curious. If it stopped hurting, why is he coming for help now? Did it really hurt at one time or did he say that so the dentist wouldn't be too disappointed?

Dentist: How long ago did it cause you pain?

Arnold: About a month and a half ago.

Dentist: Was the boil actually there when the pain was present?

Arnold: Yeah, I think so.

Comment: Really, or was this suggested to him?

Dentist: Is there any sensitivity, like to hot or cold?

Arnold: Well, it kind of hurts when I put hot things in my mouth.

Dentist: Hot liquids, like hot coffee?

Arnold: Yes. (To himself: If that's what the doc wants to hear.)

Dentist: Does it hurt when you bite down hard on something?

Arnold: (To himself: I wonder what this guy means by "hard" and by "something." It hurt when I bit a cherry seed in a pie, but that was on the other side. But I guess that qualifies for a yes answer. But why get into that?) Umm, no, not especially. (To himself: I bet this dentist guy won't even pick up on my "especially." I bet he won't even notice how I slipped in that qualifier.)

Dentist: Okay, and how long has it been since you've seen a dentist?

Arnold: (To himself: See, I thought so. He never heard it. Wonder if he was worrying about his next question rather than listening to me?) When I was in the army—during my physical.

Dentist: How long has it been since you've been out of the army?

Arnold:	About 2 years. About that, yeah. (To himself: Bet the doc doesn't realize I was in for 6 years and the only time I saw a dentist was when I enlisted.)
Dentist:	How often do you brush? Once a day? Twice a day?
Question:	What is wrong with this last question?
Answer:	The dentist said too much. What if Mr. Arnold actually brushed once a week? How could he answer "Once a day? Twice a day?" The dentist should have stopped with the question "How often do you brush your teeth?"
Arnold:	Yeah, about that.
Comment:	Now what does that mean? Once a month?
Dentist:	Okay, do you use dental floss?
Arnold:	No.
Dentist:	What kind of toothbrush do you use? Stiff? Soft?
Question:	Rephrase this last question to eliminate the suggestions.
Answer:	The dentist might have asked, "What is your toothbrush like?" or "What are the bristles like on your toothbrush?" If the patient then did not say how soft they were, the dentist could follow up with, "Are they soft, medium, or hard?" When giving a patient adjectives to describe qualities, give at least three to five choices, to avoid suggesting the answer that you expect to hear.

The following is the same interview as it might be conducted by another dentist who is perhaps more experienced or skilled.

Dentist:	Mr. Dean Arnold? Hi, I'm Dr. Arthur Drew. Please come this way with me.
Arnold:	Okay.
Dentist:	(After being seated.) What is the situation that brings you here today?
Arnold:	I've got this boil here on my gum. It's really kind of bothering me.
Dentist:	How is that?
Arnold:	Well, for a couple a months' I've noticed this lump on my gum. At first, it didn't bother me. I mean, there was no pain or anything. I just noticed it when I brushed my teeth. The brush would hit it, and it was a little tender. Then it got worse for a while, so that when I ate, it bothered me some. Occasionally, if I chewed something tough, like hard bread, it would hurt, and at times it would even bleed a little. Here lately, it hasn't hurt as much, but I'm concerned that it hasn't gone away.
Dentist:	Did hot or cold foods or drinks ever bother it?

Arnold: No, not really. But a shot of whiskey would set it on fire.

Comment: Allowing the patient to tell his story, to take responsibility, and to volunteer information provides the following benefits:
1. More information is gained per unit of time.
2. More reliable information is obtained.
3. The interviewer does not have to work nearly as hard.

Ms. Wise

a poor beginning

Dentist:	Ms. Wise?
Wise:	Yes. Dr. Cooper?
Comment:	In this instance the dentist's name is not Cooper but Curpus. It would have been much better for Dr. Curpus to have identified himself immediately rather than have the patient embarrassingly use the wrong name. He could have begun by saying: "Ms. Wise, I am Dr. Curpus. Please sit down."
Dentist:	The name is Curpus. Please sit down. Have you checked in with the secretary?
Wise:	Yes.
Dentist:	Okay, Ms. Wise, do you have any problem with your teeth?
Question:	What is wrong with this opening question?
Answer:	The question is too narrow in its focus. How would the patient respond if she were having trouble with her gums, jaw, articulation, chewing, or so on?
Question:	Make up a better opening question.
Answer:	Compare your reply with the following: What brings you to see me today? What is the situation that you have come to see me about? What can I do for you today? What troubles are you having? (A problem with this reply is its inference that the patient must have trouble before she can come to see you. Maybe she is coming for a routine checkup.) What's up? (If you know the patient and have a less formal relationship with your patients.)
Wise:	Well, I don't know; that is what I came to see you for.
Dentist:	That is what you came to see me for! Okay. Well, we'll find out. Let me take a quick history, okay? Have you been ill?

103

Question: How could you improve this reply?

Answer: There are many ways to improve this reply:

1. The dentist is the one taking responsibility for the information, but he has no need to do so. It is the patient's responsibility to give information to help himself. The dentist was doing very well until he failed to wait for the patient's response after he said, "That is what you came to see me for. . . ." At that point the dentist should have said no more. Then the patient would have had to take the responsibility.

2. What is a *quick* history? Is that a bad one? Is it incomplete? The word "quick" should have been omitted.

3. "We'll find out," sounds like a challenge or a declaration of war. "I'm going to get this history out of you, whatever it takes. I take full responsibility, and by God, you better participate."

Wise: No, I haven't been ill.

Dentist: Do you have any allergies?

Wise: Just hay fever–type allergies.

Question: What did the patient mean by this last response?

Answer: It isn't clear. The point of an interview, and the major difference between an interview and a questionnaire, is that you are spending your valuable time in the interview to *make meaning* out of what the patient says. If all you do is fill out a questionnaire for the patient, why are you doing it? Why not have a less expensive clerk do it? The dentist should have said something to the effect: "Hay fever–type allergies? Like what?"

Dentist: Okay, taking any medications?

Wise: No.

Question: How reliable is this last answer?

Answer: Not very reliable, since we have already established an adversary, competitive relationship in which yes and no answers are highly unreliable (see the section in Chapter 7 on "yes" and "no" answers, p. 52).

Dentist: We'll give you a quick examination. Do you have any tenderness under here?

Question: What is the meaning of the dentist's use of "we"?

Answer: If he is working with an assistant, "we" makes some sense. If not, the plural pronoun has the effect of depersonalizing and downgrading the dentist's responsibility. It indicates that he is not taking full responsibility for what is being done.

Wise: Well, a little bit.

Dentist: Where?

Wise:	Right under here. Feel that big ball here? What is that?
Dentist:	Ah, that's nothing, probably nothing.
Comment:	Is it nothing or probably nothing? How can the patient have any confidence when the dentist is so indefinite? It would be better for the dentist to say, "I don't know." That would be more definite than "nothing, probably nothing."
Wise:	Look, Doctor! I don't want to be told . . .
Comment:	We suggest that you role play the above with a partner. When you come to the end, continue the dialogue to its natural conclusion by making up your own lines. Pick up the mood of the person you are playing and just continue the mood to see what you can learn about the style of interacting presented in this interview.

The pedodontic office
pedodontist receptionist's challenge

Receptionist:	Dr. Frank's office, Kay speaking.
Mother:	I'm new in town, and I would like some information about your office. How much is a dental appointment?
Receptionist:	As a rule, our examination appointment is $16.00. This includes the mouth examination, cleaning the teeth, x-rays, and a fluoride treatment.
Mother:	How much is a filling?
Receptionist:	There is no set charge for a filling. After the doctor has done the mouth examination and checks the x-rays, he will give you an estimate as to how much the work will be.
Comment:	How deep is the hole, and how much time, energy, and materials will it take to fill it? How can you have a set fee for a filling of unknown dimensions?
Mother:	Does the doctor have an aid to work with him at the chair at all times?
Receptionist:	We have a dental assistant who helps the doctor when necessary. If the child is apprehensive, then the assistant is at the chair at all times.
Question:	Since we do not know what this mother is really asking, what would be a better reply to find out?
Answer:	The following are several replies the receptionist might have used to explore the mother's concerns: You seem to be concerned about that. Why do you ask? I don't know what you're really asking me. I don't understand what you want to know.

Interviews 6 through 10, relating to pedodontics, have been adapted with permission from encounters in the office of Edwin F. Froelich, D.D.S., Santa Barbara, Calif.

Comment: Some dental professionals prefer using the original reply and leaving the concerns unknown. The receptionist's response avoids the need for dealing with the concern. It may even save time at this interaction, but it may also possibly aggravate a treatment session should you plan a procedure that unknowingly triggers the mother's concern. Once again, there is no one best way to reply.

Mother: What sort of person is the doctor? The last doctor's attitude was that he didn't really care if it hurt.

Receptionist: Since you are new in town, I would suggest that you check with some of your newly acquired friends to see where they take their children. Or you might ask your own dentist or doctor for a referral.

Comment: By this statement the receptionist is suggesting that this office is in command of the situation, is willing to stand on its reputation, and is direct and open in its dealings with patients.

Mother: You were the first one to suggest that. I would like to go ahead and make an appointment with your office.

APPOINTMENTS FOR LAURIE AND PAUL

Dentist: We're going to need appointments for Laurie to treat her cavities and a broken corner of one tooth. (With that the dentist gives the receptionist the patient's card indicating the number of visits needed, the length of the visits, and the charge for the entire planned treatment.)

Receptionist: For Laurie, and that's a half hour.

Dentist: Yes, two one-half hour sessions for Laurie. I think that would be better than an hour stretch for her. (Laurie is 4 years old.)

Receptionist: Okay, and just one appointment for Paul?

Dentist: That's correct.

Receptionist: (Turning to the mother as the dentist leaves.) Is there one day that's better than another?

Mother: Thursday.

Receptionist: How about Thursday, the twentieth?

Mother: That's fine.

Receptionist: We start at 8:00, if that's any help.

Mother: We're out in the county, and that makes it kind of hard. I'll have to take the kids back out to school.

Receptionist: How would 8:30 be?

Comment: Here the receptionist is responding to the mother and reacting positively to her statement.

Mother: What does Wednesday afternoon look like? Bob plays golf on Wednesdays and could pick us up.

Receptionist: We're not here on Wednesdays.

Comment: A simple statement. The receptionist did *not* say guiltily,

"I'm sorry, but we're not here on Wednesdays." How much more comfortable it is when there is no apology!

Mother:	Well, okay, whatever. (At this point she is trapped; she gives in and will accept anything.)
Receptionist:	Then Thursday the twentieth at 8:30.
Mother:	Okay.
Receptionist:	Now, we'll need two for Laurie; the following Thursday will be the twenty-seventh.
Mother:	Okay.
Receptionist:	Okay, and then you'll bring your insurance? Well, you have a different insurance—you get your own forms—you're not insured through XYZ, are you?
Question:	This last statement is awkward. How would you rephrase the question?
Answer:	What company are you insured by? Is it XYZ?
Mother:	I'm not sure; I'll check.
Receptionist:	Let me check your card. No, you will need to get the forms from your company.
Mother:	Okay, I'll see you Thursday.
Receptionist:	Fine, see you then.

APPOINTMENTS FOR MICHELLE

Receptionist:	(On telephone.) Ms. Love?
Mother:	Yes.
Receptionist:	After checking the x-rays, Dr. Carter has found that Michelle has 14 teeth with cavities. There are 22 areas of decay.
Mother:	Oh my gosh!
Receptionist:	And the estimate on the work to be done, including her examination appointment, is $233.00.
Mother:	Two hundred and thirty-three!
Receptionist:	And she will need six appointments to get her work completed.
Comment:	The receptionist did not react to the mother's last two responses. The receptionist has a set story to tell and is continuing with it despite the mother's startled reaction.
Question:	How would you respond to this mother when she says, "Oh my gosh!" to the information about the number of cavities?
Answer:	Compare your reply with the following: You were not expecting that.

	Kind of a shock, isn't it?
	Silence. Wait for the news to sink in and for her further response. She will probably ask a question that will put the news into some kind of perspective that she can understand. At this point you don't know whether she is most interested in how much time, money, pain, or permanent disability will be involved, so let her ask for what she wants to know.
Mother:	I can't pay that to you all at once.
Comment:	Look where this mother is! She is way back on the money, and since then the receptionist has given additional information. Do you think the mother heard the information about six appointments?
Receptionist:	Well, payments on the account are just fine as long as we receive a payment each month. We have an auditor who comes in once a month to check the accounts.
Mother:	Oh, that's good. I know I can make a payment each month.
Question:	The sentence about the auditor probably wasn't heard by the mother and could have been omitted. How would you translate the sentence about the auditor?
Answer:	This sentence might be translated, "We are not mean people, but we have this nasty auditor who insists that every patient pay something every month." It is an attempt to duck the responsibility of saying, "We have instructed our auditor to see that every patient pays something every month." This sentence also implies some feelings of guilt about asking for payment for services rendered.
Receptionist:	Then may we set up an appointment?
Mother:	Fine.

INTERVIEW 8 Communicating with a four-year-old

There are many channels of communication available between two people that we use all of the time, such as touch, voice, pitch, movement, and smell (see Chapter 10). All are part of the communication from a dental professional to a patient. The following interaction between a pedodontist and a patient who is 4 years old illustrates how some of these channels are used.

Dentist: What's this little girl's name?

Kathy: Kathy.

Dentist: That's a nice name. How old are you?

Kathy: Four.

Dentist: Four years old! Let's see how many teeth you have. Oh, these are so pretty! Now see this instrument? It blows air. See it on my arm? Feel this on your hand. Well, that's going to dry the tooth so that I can see it better.

Comment: Here the pedodontist uses touch (of the air jet) to acquaint the patient with the next procedure. This is his way of telling the child what to expect next. "See what it is and how it works, so you don't have to be afraid of it." This procedure is much better than telling the child about it in words that the child would not understand and can also be used to acquaint the child with the water jet and the brush for cleaning teeth.

Dentist: Your teeth are pretty, white ones, aren't they?

Kathy: That's 'cause I brush them.

Dentist: You do. They are so pretty. Now all I have to do is polish them. I won't have to clean them. Well, let's take this little toothbrush now, and I'll show you how it works. See it spin on my thumb? Can you feel it like that? (Touching Kathy's thumb.)

Kathy: Yes!

Dentist: Good! Let's put some toothpaste in here, and then we can polish your teeth.

Comment: Another effective use of touch—to allay fear and show what will happen.

111

Advice and education

DOREEN

The patient, Doreen, is a 5½-year-old girl who has been brought to the dentist's office by her mother for a routine checkup.

Dentist: (To the patient's mother.) Your daughter is perfect. These teeth are so loose that I really couldn't clean that one. They are getting ready to come out.

Mother: Doreen, you're going to grow your big teeth.

Comment: What do the words "big teeth" mean to the patient? Something pleasant or something frightening?

Dentist: I did see one thing that may be a problem later on. (To Doreen.) Close your teeth, Doreen. Wait now, real easy. Now let me close them. Let's hold it right there. (To the mother.) These two teeth—this lower one should be in front of that upper one. So it means that the lower jaw is back in relation to the upper jaw. What we don't know at this stage of growth is whether the upper jaw is too far forward in relation to fixed points on the skull, whether the lower jaw is too far back, whether it's a combination of the two. And then, what it is, how much it is, and whether we need to do anything about it.

Comment: This last sentence could have been omitted.

Dentist: It's just something we've put down on her record card. When she gets to be about 9 or 10 years old, we'll have an orthodontist see her. For now, she's fine for 6 months. (To Doreen.) You get to go find a prize on my shelf. Go on and find one.

Comment: Nowhere in this instruction is there an opportunity for the dentist to learn what the mother understands about what is being said.

Question: How would you learn what the mother understands? What would you ask her?

Answer: Compare your answer with the following:
Do you understand? (If the mother answers yes, follow up by

saying, "Tell me what you understand so that we're in agreement.")

What is your understanding about this?

Is this clear to you?

ERIC

In the following interaction the dentist is speaking to the father of Eric, a 4-year-old boy who has a decayed tooth. The dentist wants the father to understand the problem and why something must be done about it.

Dentist: I want to show you what this decay of Eric's looks like before I remove it, and I also want to show it to you on the x-ray. You see that white area in between the teeth? That's how the cavity begins. Eventually, it destroys the tooth structure in between the teeth. There is decay over on the side. I'll show it to you when it's all uncovered. Before we uncover it, all you can see is a little tiny spot. When I get finished with this, I'll show you the x-ray and the whole thing. Okay?

Father: Okay.

Dentist: Very good! I'll show it to you later.

Comment: We are salespeople. We must sell patients on what we know will be of benefit to their health and happiness. Part of this selling involves educating them so that they understand what we want them to do, participate in, and pay for. Showing them the x-ray film, the unprepared tooth, the prepared cavity, and the finished product are all part of the selling. As with all selling, you may lose the client if you talk down to him/her.

Question: How can you avoid talking down to the patient and the patient's parent as you show them the x-ray film?

Answer: You must first find out how much they can see on their own.

Question: How would you proceed after the following: "I want to show you what this decay looks like before I remove it, and I also want to show it to you on the x-ray . . . "

Answer: Can you see the decay on this tooth? (You might be surprised when the patient says yes and points it out. When the patient says no, you have lost nothing and have avoided the possibility of talking down to the patient.)

Hygienist's instructions

Hygienist:	Hi Amy, how are you?
Amy:	Hello. (Amy is 15 years old.)
Hygienist:	You're here for your regular checkup?
Amy:	Uh huh.
Hygienist:	Gee, how long has it been?
Amy:	I don't know.
Hygienist:	Let's check the chart. It looks like you were in 13 months ago. Let's take a look and see how things are. Well, your teeth look good, just from looking at them, Amy, but you may have some plaque on them. It's invisible; you can't see it. So maybe we should stain them and see if we can see any plaque, because plaque is very harmful for your gums.
Comment:	It would be better to omit the "So maybe . . . " and just begin with "We should . . . "
Hygienist:	It makes them sore, and they may bleed. It also causes cavities. So it's best if we stain your teeth and see if you do have any plaque.
Amy:	What's it from?
Hygienist:	Bacteria, mainly; it's also from the food you eat. It produces an acid, and that's when decay happens. So it's important that we remove the plaque, and we'll be doing that today by cleaning your teeth. Then I'll teach you how to keep it off of your teeth by brushing and using dental floss. First, let's have you look in the mirror and see if you can see any plaque without the stain.
Amy:	Huh uh, I can't see anything.
Hygienist:	They look fine, don't they? Run your tongue over them. Do they feel a little furry, a little grimy?

Adapted with permission from a session conducted by Marlene Taylor, M.S., in the office of
Edwin F. Froelich, D.D.S., Santa Barbara, Calif.

Amy:	A little bit.
Question:	The meaning of Amy's answer is anyone's guess. Does the answer mean that the patient is being agreeable? Rephrase the hygienist's question.
Answer:	Run your tongue over them. What do they feel like?
Hygienist:	Well, that's probably plaque that you feel. As I said, you can't see it, but you can feel it with your tongue.
Amy:	When does it start, like if I don't brush?
Hygienist:	If you don't brush, it will form within 24 hours. You can have a new organization of plaque. It forms in little clumps, and if you don't disturb the clumping with a toothbrush or dental floss, it can cause decay and sore gums. So every 24 hours you should thoroughly remove the plaque from your mouth.
Amy:	What happens if you don't?
Hygienist:	If you don't it can become tartar, for one thing; and I think you have a little bit of that. It can become calcified, and then it becomes tarter; that begins within 48 hours. Also, as I said, if you don't disturb the organization of plaque within 24 hours, you can have a cavity. It can start to decay your tooth because of the acid that it produces.
Amy:	Can you get the tarter off?
Hygienist:	You can't, but I can. You have to visit your dentist or dental hygienist to remove the tarter from your teeth, because it's hard. But the plaque you can remove at home. Now let's stain your teeth; then we'll look with the plaque light. All right, now swish that around in your mouth. When it's all around, over all the surfaces, empty it out.
Amy:	Is this like that red stuff they have on commercials?
Hygienist:	Yes. This is different, but it does the same thing. Now that you have rinsed, Amy, let's look with the plaque light. There you go. Now see what you can see in your mouth.
Amy:	Right there in that little hole—in front of the tooth.
Hygienist:	Uh huh, you have plaque there.
Amy:	Why do I have that little hole there in the front of that tooth?
Hygienist:	That's a defect in your tooth. Your tooth came in like that.
Amy:	(Laughing.) Ah, oh my tongue.
Hygienist:	Stick your tongue out. See the plaque?
Amy:	Is it important to brush your tongue, too?
Hygienist:	Yes. Now look all around on the inside, next to your tongue.

That's a common area for people to miss when they brush. See in there, right along the gum line; you missed this area with your toothbrush today. Here in front you are pretty good; look around, mostly you've missed gum line areas, and that's where most people do miss.

Amy: And in between my teeth.

Hygienist: Yes. Your toothbrush should be effective at the gum line, and the dental floss is effective in between your teeth. Now you look around; I want you to remember the places where we see that you have the most trouble getting the plaque, so that you can concentrate on them when you brush.

Amy: Why do you use this type of light?

Hygienist: Well, this type of light works on the yellow and makes it fluorescent somehow. If you just stained your teeth with this, you wouldn't see the plaque. You have to shine the light on it.

Amy: It's funny they would use something that you need a special light for.

Hygienist: We can give you some red tablets to use at home. I'll give you instructions on how you can use them the same way. I used this method just now because it's a little more dramatic. It shows up the plaque better.

Amy: And with the red tablets I can check at home.

Hygienist: Right. Let's go ahead now, Amy, and clean your teeth.

Comment: Note how the hygienist replied to each of Amy's questions. The hygienist was really listening.

LATER

Hygienist: Okay, we're all done cleaning. Let's see, now that I've removed the plaque by cleaning your teeth, let's restain and use the plaque light again. Okay, now rinse it out. We always rinse this off so that what stain is left is on the plaque. Great. Now let's look again to see if I've done my job.

Amy: I don't see anything.

Hygienist: I see just a tiny bit. I'll have to go back and clean it.

Amy: Yeah, right there. And there's a place on my front tooth, too.

Hygienist: Yeah, you're going to have to watch that when you're brushing, because it's a source for collecting plaque, which could eventually decay that spot for you. But if you keep it clean, it should be all right.

Amy: I love having my teeth clean.

Hygienist: Yeah, well, now you are going to be able to keep them that way, because I'm going to show you how to remove the plaque.

They should feel just like they feel right now, every day. It's sort of hard, though, to remove all of the plaque; that's why people keep coming to the dentist; we don't all have that much dexterity. Okay, now let's see. Let's start with the toothbrushing. Do you have a soft toothbrush at home?

Amy: It's a medium, I think. I don't like soft ones.

Hygienist: You don't like soft ones?

Comment: A good reflection to get Amy to elaborate.

Amy: I don't feel like they clean my teeth.

Hygienist: A whole lot of people say that, Amy. So what you could do to satisfy me is to use your old toothbrush for the way you're brushing now, and I'll give you the name of the one I want you to get for a special way of brushing that I'm going to show you today. This new way of brushing will get your teeth clean, but they may not feel like it, because of something different.

Comment: The hygienist has let herself open to having the patient act out against her should the patient get angry. She told the patient to get a new, soft brush to satisfy her, the hygienist, rather than to take better care of the patient's teeth. This technique in patient management is a risky one.

Amy: Why do you need a soft toothbrush?

Hygienist: Well, because you're going to use it at the gum line. A stiffer brush would possibly injure your gums. The other reason is that a soft, dry toothbrush traps plaque. These soft bristles are made to remove the plaque. You're not going to use toothpaste or water when you brush, because they interfere with the removal of plaque.

Amy: What about when you're brushing, like on your teeth, does the hard toothbrush push more . . .

Hygienist: No, a hard toothbrush can cause what we call erosion. It can actually wear your teeth away if you're a vigorous brusher. But it's all right to do that here on the chewing surfaces, like so. That's fine. You can scrub on the chewing surfaces, but along the gum line is where you don't want to actually use scrubbing.

Amy: Why is that toothbrush shaped funny?

Hygienist: This one is curved to conform better to your mouth. This is for a right-handed person, and it's bent here so that when you are brushing with your right hand, it gets to the left side of your mouth better. You see, this is where people are very . . .

Amy: What about when you get to the other side?

Hygienist: Well, the other side is easier for a right-handed person to get to, so that isn't the problem. You don't have the problem on your right side that you do on your left, so that's why this one is bent.

For a left-handed person, you bend it the other way. You can bend your own, maybe by heating it up first. Okay, now what we're going to do with the brushing is something you probably haven't done before. We're going to place the bristles way down, right at the gum line, like this. The pointed end right in here. This is called the surface. This is where plaque starts to grow, so we're going to attack it right at its source. Then we're going to use pressure, a gentle pressure, and jiggle these bristles, like this. Okay, now we're going to go all around. It's important to start in one area and finish the whole outside of your teeth. Don't skip from spot to spot. Have a routine when you brush so that you don't miss anything. Okay, after you finish the outside, get the brush on the inside in the same fashion, using pressure and jiggling. Until you get here (in front), this brush does not fit across here, and yours will not, either. Tip the brush up on end. You may have been doing this with your regular brushing. Make circles and come out like so, just for this area. This method cleans this area best. Now return to the pressure and jiggling motion. Hold the brush like a pencil. Does it feel weird to brush this way?

Amy:　Yeah.

Hygienist:　Well, try it, because this way prevents you from doing what we call cross brushing, like this. If you're jiggling across, you'll have a tendency to do that. If you're holding it this other way, as much as you possibly can, you won't have the tendency as much. So remember, the brush head stays in one spot, and you just jiggle the bristles. Okay, we're finished the lower jaw. It's the same thing on the upper jaw, only these bristles are pointed up into the gum line, just underneath, with the same pressure and jiggling motion. Again, start in one spot and finish all the way around, doing the same thing up here. Again, what happens up here? You'll have to turn the brush up on end and make circles again. Now, as I said, this is done with no toothpaste or water once a day, but this doesn't mean that you shouldn't also brush with a fluoride toothpaste. You should.

Amy:　Does it matter what time of day I brush my teeth?

Hygienist:　No, it doesn't matter—whatever time you get your habit going. It should be habit forming—a pattern and a habit. You can brush in the morning after breakfast or at night before you go to bed. After you've used the dry brush, you could put toothpaste on and finish brushing, or you could finish brushing with the toothbrush that you like. Well, at any rate, don't go home and use your harder bristle brush like the way I just showed you, or you'll do some injury. Well, that pretty well takes care of brushing your teeth on all the surfaces, but in between . . .

Amy:　What about mouthwash?

Hygienist:　Any mouthwash is fine.

Amy:	'Cause I, the other thing I've heard is that it kills the good bacteria in your mouth.
Hygienist:	I don't think that you have to worry about that. You do have to remember that it really doesn't do anything for you as far as removing bad breath is concerned. It masks it. It doesn't generally remove the bacteria. Your brushing and flossing remove the bacteria, so you can be confident that you don't have bad breath if you're doing a super job of brushing and flossing.
Amy:	What about using baking soda instead of toothpaste?
Hygienist:	That's fine.
Amy:	Does it have the fluoride?
Hygienist:	No. I would say not instead of, but in addition to, toothpaste.
Amy:	But, don't we get fluoride in our water?
Hygienist:	We do have some fluoride in some parts of the city here. I think you probably do in your area, but it's still important to use the fluoride.
Amy:	Any toothpaste?
Hygienist:	Probably any one of the fluorides, but your baking soda is okay, too, if you want to add that to the toothpaste. Okay, now this is the part that . . .
Amy:	Like Ultra Brite, is that, does that have fluoride in it?
Hygienist:	No. Ultra Brite's all right if, well, if you're using fluoride too, you see. The thing that we want to get across is that everybody should use fluoride. Now, when you use dental floss— I'll give you this to take home. Take a big piece of it off; be generous. You can't floss with just a little piece like this. You're going to wrap it around your fourth finger, like this, on each hand. Holding this is just as important as flossing, because you do a better job if you're holding it right. Hold this nice and tight here and use these two fingers to floss with. I'll show you, then I'll let you try it. These fingers should be close together, because if they get apart, like this, you'll find that you've lost control of the dental floss. Now, this dental floss is not just to remove food from in between your teeth. That's how most people have used it in the past, but you're supposed to slide it down the tooth, like this, to clean the tooth's surface (using a model). You go way down under there—see how far down the tooth— like this, and clean the tooth's surface. You go way down under there—see how far down I've gone—and then straight up, like this. Come up over that tissue and get down here and scrape up, like so, and pop it out, like this. But the two important things for you to remember when you do it are not to go in down straight on that tissue—that would cut it—and when you get down here,

	don't go straight across. Come up over the tissue. When you get to the back teeth, remember that the tissue in between all of your teeth is knife-like, so that you have to come in over that. The way I suggest, though, when you're learning to use dental floss, is to floss from this cuspid to this cuspid on your lowers and from this cuspid to this cuspid on your uppers, so that you'll get the feel and learn where it's easiest. Then add the back teeth. Do it this way. When you get good at this, you can do it while you're watching television.
Amy:	Okay.
Hygienist:	You probably spend some time in front of the television. But at first, you'll need to use a mirror. I've found that other people sometimes don't want to spend extra time in the bathroom, but eventually you could use your floss or even your toothbrush, if you're using it dry, while you're studying if you have a lot of homework to do.
Amy:	That sounds more realistic to me.
Hygienist:	Okay, want to try it now? I'll just let you take off with some of this, and I'll hold the mirror for you. Okay, does that feel comfortable? That's a little far apart; see if you can get it closer together. Your teeth are close together, Amy. See, you're going to have some trouble. Try to follow that tooth down and not snap the floss in. Good, you're not going to have too much trouble at all. You seem to be able to do it. Are you getting down underneath the gum line? That's the important part. Now, for awhile you'll find that your gums will be sore after you do this, and they may bleed; but don't give up. That's just normal. After a while they'll get real tough, and it won't be uncomfortable anymore. Now, you're going to have some trouble where you saw the plaque on these uppers. Remember, you'll have to try to get up and around in there, too. In fact, it may be easier. They're a little further apart. Okay, you look like you've used dental floss before, Amy.
Amy:	Uh huh.
Hygienist:	Good. That's unwaxed dental floss that I'm giving you.
Amy:	Does it matter?
Hygienist:	The unwaxed is a little finer, and it does tend to cut through the plaque better than the waxed.
Amy:	Especially with my teeth being so close together.
Hygienist:	But if you find that you have trouble with this unwaxed floss breaking off, you might try the waxed kind.
Amy:	Okay, fine.
Hygienist:	But I think you're going to be all right. You're getting to where you don't need to look in the mirror, already. All right, just

	remember to keep your fingers wrapped and keep them close together.
Amy:	I'm going to cut off the circulation to my poor fingers.
Hygienist:	I'll show you a better way to hold it. That first way is about the easiest way I can show anyone, but there's a better way to hold it. It's like this.
Amy:	Yeah, that's what I usually do.
Hygienist:	Somebody has already shown you that.
Comment:	The hygienist would have saved a lot of time if she had established early whether the patient had used dental floss before, how she held it, how she used it, and so on. Why teach a college student the basic math tables if the student has already mastered them and gone beyond?
Amy:	That feels natural.
Hygienist:	Good. that's good, because it's sort of hard for most people to pick up on the first visit, but that's the way it's done, like that. Good. Okay, well, I guess that just about does it.
Amy:	Great.
Hygienist:	For 6 months. I'll have the doctor examine your mouth. We've taken x-rays today, and you won't need to return for 6 months.
Amy:	Great. Thanks so much.
Hygienist:	Okay, see you then.

Original examination of an orthodontic patient

Dentist:	You are 9 years old; is that right, Martha?
Martha:	Yes.
Dentist:	Do you have regular dental checkups?
Question:	What does "regular dental checkups" mean to a 9-year-old? What is a better way of asking for this information?
Answer:	Compare your answer with the following: How often have you been to a dentist? Have you been to a dentist before? How long has it been since you've gone to a dentist?
Martha:	Yes.
Dentist:	Do you brush your teeth at home?
Martha:	Yes.
Question:	What information would you now want to have?
Answer:	Remember, the purpose of an interview is to follow up and make meaning out of what the patient says. Thus, the most important next step is to make meaning out of the patient's last answer by asking how, and how often, she brushes her teeth.
Dentist:	How often do you brush your teeth?
Martha:	Every night.
Dentist:	Good. (Turning to the patient's mother.) How about her tonsils and adenoids?
Mother:	She had a tonsillectomy, and I can't tell you if they took her adenoids out or not.

Interviews 11 and 12 have been adapted with permission from encounters in the office of John S. Rathbone, D.D.S., Santa Barbara, Calif.

Dentist:	I asked that because we're interested in her airway passage. Does she have any allergies?
Mother:	No, none that I know of.
Dentist:	Very good. (To Martha.) Well, it looks like you're in very good health. Let's take a look at your teeth. (To the mother.) Martha's primary problem is what we consider a very deep overbite. Her upper teeth go way down over her lower teeth. She also has a problem of alignment with her upper teeth. Her lower teeth have good alignment. She still has two baby teeth on the lower, and four on the upper. If you'll notice her face pattern, she has a real good chin, a real good angle of her jaw—the larger this angle becomes, the more it drops the chin down and back. She has a very straight face, so I would say from a preliminary examination that she is going to have plenty of room in her mouth for all of her permanent teeth. The big question is just opening her bite. She has no difficulty in closing her lips. When we complete orthodontic treatment, we would like to have her lips close together so as not to have any of the facial muscles tighten up. Because she has such a good angle and plenty of room for all of her permanent teeth, my suggestion to you would be to wait until she has all of her permanent teeth before we do any treatment. Martha is almost 10 years old?
Mother:	Yes.
Dentist:	We probably won't treat her for at least a year or a year and a half. Then we will start her treatment.
Mother:	How do you do this?
Dentist:	She's going to need a full hookup of bands or braces. (To Martha.) What do they call them at school?
Comment:	This question to the child brings her back into the conversation and encourages her continued participation, listening, and learning.
Martha:	Braces.
Dentist:	By waiting until she has all of her permanent teeth, we can do all of her treatment at one time or in one stage.
Mother:	How do you open the bite?
Dentist:	We have to depress the front teeth and elongate the back teeth, and this we can do very easily, but it's going to take braces or bands on all of her permanent teeth.
Mother:	The front ones should be aligned, and you won't push them back at all?
Dentist:	We will align all of her front teeth and retract her upper teeth a little. Basically, her teeth go together very well in back. She has a little bit of protrusion. This is all done together. What

I'm saying is that yes, she has a problem. There is a correct time to treat it. I think with her type of problem, where she has such a good face pattern and plenty of room for all of her teeth and where it is just a question of opening her bite, reducing a little bit of protrusion, and aligning her teeth, we should wait for all of her permanent teeth. I think she will need to have braces for about 20 to 22 months. After we take the braces off, she will wear a retainer until her wisdom teeth are in place or, if necessary, removed. We are interested in stability just as much as we are in tooth alighment. We are hoping to align these teeth so that if Martha takes care of them, they should last her until she is 80 years old.

Mother: Can you give me some idea of the cost?

Dentist: Yes. Basically, we work on a set fee, and you can determine how you would like to pay it or what fits into your budget. I can't be specific at this time, but the fee will be approximately $1,300 to $1,400 for the complete treatment including the retainers.

Mother: Thank you. Now, will you contact us when you want to see Martha?

Dentist: Yes. We will place Martha in our recall system and notify you in 1 year. Are there any other questions?

Mother: No. We will wait to hear from you. Goodbye.

Comment: This consultation demonstrates an example of simple, direct, open communication between the dentist, the patient, and her mother. The mother had the opportunity to ask questions and clarify what she did not understand, as did the dentist. He obtained a minimal history sufficient for his consultation. He also conveyed sufficient information for the mother to feel that she understood what needed to be done.

Establishing a long-term contract

Although this interview deals with orthodontics, our intent is to focus on the process of establishing a long-term contract.

Interview 11 shows how an orthodontist might handle a consultation in which treatment would not be started for 1 or 2 years. The diagnostic evaluation has already been completed for the patient in this interview, and in this session the dentist is establishing the contract for treatment with the patient's mother. (For this type of session, both parents may be present.)

While reading this interview, consider the pathways of communication. Who is the patient? With whom is the dental contract made? With whom is the legal contract made? How old should a patient be before you make the contract with the patient? What is your dental contract with a minor? What expectations, obligations, responsibilities, and agreements must a young patient make with you, the dental professional, for your treatment to be successful? We have no definitive answers; these must come from you.

Dentist: (To the patient's mother.) These are the models, photographs, and x-ray films of Mike's teeth and head. This is the supplementary tracing of the lateral head x-ray that we had taken at the laboratory. We use this tracing because it gives us a chance to compare him with a large group of young people as to how his teeth fit together in relation to his jaw and to the rest of his head. Basically, there are four things that interest us. The first thing we're interested in is lip closure and profile. We would like to have the lips come together at the folds so that when they're completely relaxed, they just fall together. Actually Mike's problem isn't too bad. He's full in the lips because of his deep overbite, and he has too much curl to his lower lip. We would like to flatten his lips so that the amount of curl in the lower lip is reduced.

    The second thing we're interested in is basic tooth alignment. There's no problem in Mike's arch form. He's got good, acceptable tooth alignment. In the lower front he does have some minor jumbling, but it's very minor. He does have spaces in the back, so he has plenty of room for all of his permanent teeth.

    The third thing we're interested in is the functional aspect of how his teeth go together in terms of how one jaw fits in relation to the other. How they fit in the back and whether he has a deep overbite. His front-back relationship is correct, but he does have a deep overbite. I think if we allowed Mike to continue as he is, the overbite would continue to get deeper as he got older, and the result would be that eventually his lower teeth would be biting into the palate or the roof of his mouth just in back of the upper front teeth. This is the big reason why I recommend treating him.

The fourth thing we're interested in is stability. In other words, if we're going to spend money to fix Mike's teeth, we would like to align them in such a way that they're supported from one arch to the other, then if he takes care of them, they should last until he is 80 years old. For instance, if we didn't correct the alignment or if we didn't correct the overbite, as these teeth got further over each other, he could develop more of a periodontal problem; that is, the teeth might not develop adequate gum and bone support to keep them around for a long time, and this is what we want to avoid.

So these are the four things that we would like to treat Mike for: to improve his lip closure, to help him with his tooth alignment, to correct his overbite, and to improve his stability so that his teeth will last his lifetime.

Comment: After such a long, unbroken explanation it is a good procedure to make a summary statement before going any further.

Question: What is the next thing the dentist should say to the mother?

Answer: Since the most important part of a message is in the receiver, the dentist should now ask the mother if she understands what she has been told.

Question: Why isn't the patient included in the original consultation with the parent(s)?

Answer: Sometimes the patient is. It depends on the availability of the parent(s) and child at the same time. In most cases the child is not present, because in the discussion such things as finances or other family problems that would indicate a delay in treatment might arise. In addition, we have found it advisable to have a separate consultation with the child so that the child can ask his/her own questions and not be dominated by the parent(s) and so that we can explain to the child his/her responsibilities in the treatment procedures.

You might wish to consider whether the above information should have been presented to Mike at this same time rather than in a separate session. Remember, there is margin for hearing and interpreting information differently, even with the same setting. Will Mike wonder what the dentist told his mother that was not told to him? Where does telling the mother first, without Mike, place the primary responsibility for carrying out treatment? Is this a possible setup for Mike and his mother to fight about what each thinks Mike is supposed to do in following the instructions? We lean toward including the patient in every way possible as an equal, responsible party. We will continue the session with the assumption that the dentist has clarified any questions or misinformation the mother has presented.

Dentist: I notice from the health chart that he has never had his tonsils or adenoids removed. Does he have problem breathing or with allergies?

Mother: In the past he has had a little tonsillitis, where the doctor would watch him closely to see about taking them out. During this past year, though, he hasn't had any problem.

Dentist: This is one of the things that we may want to watch. As you see, he has rather narrow areas here (on the x-ray film) in the nasal passage, and what you see here on the outline could be adenoid tissue. Now you can't completely count on the x-ray, but you can get a good indication. We want him to breathe through his nose and not his mouth, so we've got to have a clear airway space. As far as the rest of the x-ray, he's developing his third molars here. He has a very good angle to his jaw and presents a good chin. He has plenty of room in his mouth for all of his teeth. He has a very clean mouth and good bone structure. The roots are well formed, and his wisdom teeth, as we pointed out, are forming. The only thing that we can't be sure of is the left upper third molar. His upper right and left cuspids have not yet erupted. We may, before we put his bands on, want to have these baby teeth removed to uncover these cuspids and facilitate the eruption of the permanent teeth so that we won't be delayed in treatment.

Comment: This is another point where the dentist should clear up any misunderstandings and answer any questions.

Dentist: Going back to the tracing of the head plate, we can see how much and how far he goes down on his overbite. He has, when we measure the point from here, what we call the A and B difference; he has a difference of 6 degrees. We would like to see a 2-degree difference. So, in treating him, we're going to do a little shifting. We're going to give him a little stronger chin, get this tooth clear up to there, reduce that protrusion, and increase his vertical height to reduce the curl in his lower lip. (Turning to a set of models showing the bands on the teeth.) I will have certain responsibilities, and Mike will have certain responsibilities. I can set up the mechanics, but unless Mike helps by wearing the headgear and elastics and by keeping his teeth clean, we may run into problems. We will be asking Mike to help us reduce the protrusion by wearing a headgear. We'll ask him to put it on after dinner at night and wear it until breakfast or for approximately 12 hours.

Comment: We are back to the idea of Mike's ultimate responsibility for the success of the treatment plan, but as we have explained, this responsibility will be brought out in a separate consultation with Mike.

Mother: Then he won't have to wear it all the time?

Comment: This is the first time the mother has taken the initiative to ask a question. Note that it is a brief question for clarification of something specific and comparatively nontechnical. It may be that wearing the headgear in public is an important issue to the mother or that she is tired of being still for so long. After all, everyone likes to say a few words now and then. At any rate, the dentist picks up on wearing the headgear in public.

Dentist: No, he won't have to wear it all the time—not during the daytime. I don't want him to be embarrassed by it. He is to wear it just in front of his immediate family. If he consciously wears it 12 to 14 hours every night, we can achieve the success that we want. Then, the other thing that Mike will be doing will be wearing elastic bands from a point up here to a point down there. Mike will have to remember to take these off for meals and then put them on again afterward. He will need to wear these all the time. So, he will wear the headgear at night and the elastics inside of his mouth all the time. Naturally, with all this hardware in his mouth, he will have difficulty brushing and keeping his teeth clean. We'll show him how to brush his teeth, talk to him about sugar intake, and teach him how to care for his teeth, in general.

Mother: He drinks root beer. That's full of sugar, isn't it?

Dentist: Yes, there's a lot of sugar in soft drinks. We would prefer that he drink dietetic ones. Of course, you have to remember that root beer passes by the teeth pretty quickly. The effect of sugar is strictly a local action. It's the collecting of the sugar in the form of plaque on the teeth that does the harm. And with braces on, it becomes even more important to keep the teeth clean. I would be more concerned about candy—candy bars, things that are sticky. In other words, peanut butter by itself is all right; when you put jelly with it, though, you have a sticky substance that contains sugar. Cookies are bad because they're sticky. A soft drink is bad, but it's not as bad as a cookie, because it passes by the teeth quickly. So, you not only have to think about the amount of sugar in the substance and the stickiness of the substance, you also have to think about how much time it's in the mouth.

We have visual aids with some good examples on film that we'll show Mike to help him learn to care for his teeth. An advantage that I have is that I'll be seeing him on a routine basis, every 3 or 4 weeks, over about 2 years. I'll be constantly encouraging him to do a good job. We find that young people are very good in taking care of their teeth. When you come down to it, there is no point in having straight teeth if you don't take care of them. These are the things that we'll discuss with Mike before we go into treatment, so that he knows exactly what his responsibilities are, what our responsibilities are, and what we expect of him. As far as soreness is concerned, he's going to feel like he has a lot of meat caught between his teeth; it's going to be a tight feeling, and it will be strange at first. It's like putting on a new pair of glasses or a new pair of shoes. We won't put all the bands on at one time. We'll put them on gradually, within a period of 3 to 4 weeks, and we'll use this time to become acquainted with Mike. We'll have him here for an hour, and we'll put on just as many as it's convenient to put on in an hour without rushing. It's Mike's first experience with getting braces, and we don't want it to be unpleasant. Again, I'll need his cooperation.

After we make a change in the arch wire, as you see here, we'll put a new wire in, and his teeth will begin moving; they're going to be sore. One of the ways to take out the soreness is to chew gum—sugarless gum. We'll give him some gum, and we'll ask him to chew it. It keeps everything in function, keeping a good blood supply. We find that this reduces the soreness. The pain threshold or tolerance is different in each patient. If Mike's sensitive, we'll just do the same job in a longer period of time and go a little slower. We can tell that at an early stage in treatment. So, we really shouldn't have any problems from the standpoint of soreness or pain. Once in a while a wire will stick him. Have him come in, and we'll fix it. Once in a while he will complain of sore teeth and won't want to eat. You may have to alter his food a little to something that isn't quite so hard to chew. I would like to know it if he has frequent problems with soreness and eating.

Our plan of treatment is going to take about 22 to 24 months. We would like to treat him during the junior high period so that when he goes into high school, he will be all through with braces. Mike is 13 and in the seventh grade; if we start him this summer, he should be all through before he enters high school. Then he won't have to worry about braces from the standpoint of social activities or athletics.

After we take the bands off, at the end of 20 to 24 months, we'll put him on retainers. The lower retainer will be a fixed one. It will be cemented on. The upper retainer will be a removable retainer. It's made of acrylic and fits into the roof of the mouth, and there is a wire around the teeth. We will ask him to wear the upper one all of the time for about 6 months, and then he will wear it less. We will probably watch him until he graduates from high school. In other words, until he is about 17. We want to follow him until after his wisdom teeth are in place or until after they have been extracted if that becomes necessary.

Comment: This information has been a lot for the mother to assimilate, but the dentist is using visual aids to explain the various procedures. Some parents respond more than others, and at this point (if not before) the dentist should check with the mother as to whether she is still following what is being told to her. We have no information here about the nonverbal signals of understanding that are being exchanged. Either the mother is indicating understanding or giving no distress signals, or the dentist is failing to notice the distress. The continued discussion by the dentist indicates that he feels Mike's mother is following what is being said.

Dentist: From a financial standpoint, we work on a set fee that takes care of everything that we'll be doing from the time that we first saw him until we're through with him. We're talking about $1,350. You can break this down any way that you want. We would prefer that you tell us how you would like the financial arrangements to be made. We would suggest that this be over a period of 2 or 2½ years, during the time that we're working on his teeth. Some people prefer to pay an initial payment of two, three or four hundred dollars; others want to do it on a straight monthly basis; some do it on a quarterly basis because they don't want monthly statements. We have others who do it on a yearly basis because if they pay it off in 1 year, it's deductible under medical expenses.

Comment: Talking about finances is like talking about death. We use nonspecific words such as "this" and "do it" to avoid emotionally charged words such as "pay," "owe," or "payment."

Mother: What about interest?

Dentist: There's no interest connected with it.

Mother: Well, that's good. I've worked with interest too long. I'm against it. But there are times when you have to pay it.

Dentist: You must remember that we're projecting treatment over a 2-year period. We're going to be spending more time in the beginning, on the models, diagnostic work, and bands, and this is the reason we can justify an initial payment. However, we find that most people are better able to meet their financial obligations when they elect their own method of payment. We don't charge any interest, because treatment extends over a 2-year period; we ask the fee be paid within this time and not to extend over 30 months. There will be no additional charges unless Mike gets very careless with his retainer, the one that is removable. We expect him to break one or two; if he gets to breaking it weekly, then we'll have to charge for it.

Mother: That certainly sounds very fair, unusually fair for these days.

Dentist: This is the middle of April. We ought to start him sometime between now and next September. It will probably be the middle of May before we can start him. At the beginning of May you might talk to Mike about our plans and tell him that we want to consult with him. In the meantime I would like to see him at least once to check on that upper cuspid. My secretary will call you about setting up the appointments ahead of time so that once we start to put his bands on, he will have enough appointments to get all the bands placed. We'll send you a letter giving us consent to treat Mike because he's a minor, and we'll outline the financial arrangements in the letter so that you can refer to it for income tax purposes. I think that people who go into orthodontic treatment know they're assuming a large financial obligation. Since treatment is over a period of time, you may elect your own method of payment.

Mother: I would rather just go ahead and start making you monthly payments by putting it into my budget now.

Dentist: Just let us know what is convenient for you. So, that's about the story of Mike's treatment. We want to help him in the four areas, lip closure, tooth alignment, function, and stability. The big factor is cooperation. We are going to work with him on that because we need his help. I don't think he should have any pain or discomfort. It's going to feel funny, but it shouldn't be so uncomfortable that he will be complaining all the time. It shouldn't stop him from any activities. It's just a question of going in and doing it. Do you have any questions?

Mother: No, I believe I understand it and will be looking for your letter.

Dentist: Fine. I'll get it to you in the next week.

Comment: Should the patient have been present during this session? Should both parents have been present? Should all of the information be summarized in a pamphlet and used to reinforce the learning and transfer of information? What does the mother really understand? Some of these questions have been brought up earlier in this interview. They are all questions to be answered individually. Each orthodontic consultation is different depending on the type of patient problem. Also, the consultation will vary from office to office depending on the orthodontist. In most cases the orthodontist attempts to keep from being too technical; yet he must present the problem (malocclusion), how it is to be treated, the responsibilities of the doctor and the patient, the fee for the services, and the options for payment. Therefore, the rather lengthy explanation by the orthodontist is necessary. In most cases the orthodontist allows 20 to 30 minutes for the consultation with the parent(s).

Introduction to appendixes

These appendixes have several functions. Appendix A provides the student (or anyone who is interested in improving his/her interacting skills) with exercises to work through for additional practice in the basic interactional principles presented in this text. These exercises may also be used by the dental professional teacher who may use them as a guide for developing his/her own exercises to fit more precisely the needs of his/her individual students.

Appendix B serves as a guide for learning through the videotaping of an interaction with a real or programmed (role-playing) patient. The interview worksheet and the interview assessment form aid in the analysis of the interaction. The worksheet is for the interviewer him/herself to use with a recording of his/her interaction. The assessment form is for an observer to use while observing the live or recorded interaction.

Appendix C provides videotape simulations, which work very well as learning vehicles in both undergraduate and continuing education settings. They aid learning by requiring close observation of the process and content of an interaction.

From the material in these appendixes the teacher can find aids for his/her next course dealing with professional interactions in the dental office, the student can find additional exercises, and the dental professional may have a more meaningful continuing education program at the next meeting.

Communication exercises

Statements made in the second and third person may frequently be blaming or accusative. That is, the receiver of the message feels that he/she is being blamed or accused of something. The receiver then becomes defensive. In the professional relationship it is rare that effective (in the sense of helping the patient grow or overcome illness) communication results from putting the patient on the defensive. The following exercise is on rephrasing second- and third-person statements into first-person statements. When a speaker makes a statement in the first person ("I think . . ." or "I feel . . ."), the speaker is taking responsibility for the statement instead of being accusative.

In the following exercise read each situation and the "you" message. Then write a clear "I" message in the third column. When you have finished, compare your "I" messages with our suggestions.

Situation	"You" message	"I" message
Example: The assistant has just reported that a patient refused to restrict his diet to liquids last night. Since the restriction was crucial to the treatment of the patient, you are concerned and puzzled.	What's the matter with you? Why didn't you avoid chewing last night?	I feel puzzled and concerned (that I was not sensitive to your feelings) about your chewing last night.
A. As a dental professional, you take a chance and choose to work with a professor who is not well-liked by other students or faculty members. Surprisingly, you find your experience to be pleasing and profitable.	It turns out that you are an impressive professor, after all.	

| B. | The hygienist corrects you regarding a procedural error that endangers a patient's tooth. | You are overstepping your bounds; would you please stop riding me? |
| C. | A patient seems to be in a depressed mood for the entire appointment. She acts very sad. | What has been the matter with you this last half hour? |

Answer: Any response is appropriate *if it begins with an "I" statement that communicates how "I feel."*

A. I feel very pleased and relieved to have worked with you this summer. It makes me feel proud to see you doing so well.

B. I feel embarrassed; I'm glad you made me aware of the error.

C. I feel worried about your sadness right now. Is there some way I can help?

Or simply: I feel concerned about your sadness right now.

THE LATENT CONTENT

A message usually has both a manifest and a latent content. The manifest content is the dictionary meaning of the words. The latent content is made up of the feelings—the inferred and understood message. When interacting with another person, we may choose to react to the manifest or latent content of each message as it is sent.

In the following exercise read each patient's statement and write a *reflection* to the latent content in the column under *Receiver (dental professional)*. When you have finished, compare your responses with ours.

Sender (patient)	**Receiver (dental professional)**
Example: This thing has been going on for weeks. I just can't go on any longer (tears). I must find some way out.	You're completely exhausted; you're at the end of your rope, and you feel that you've got to find a way out.
A. Well, what about the average person who has something like what I've got, this peridontal disease? Doesn't the surgery hurt? Won't this problem come back on me, anyway?	
B. I just wish someone would tell me what usually happens with the average patient who has been here with this disease.	
C. My mommy told me to come here by myself today.	

Answer: A. You're feeling anxious and apprehensive about the discomfort you will experience, and you wonder whether the treatment is worth it.

B. You feel irritated because we're unable to give you an answer at this time.

C. You're feeling afraid, and you wish that your mother were here.

RESTATEMENT

The use of a restatement (reflection or summary reply) in the receiving of a message can serve several purposes:

1. It can serve as an *echo* to the sender (patient) and may help the patient to continue speaking and examining his/her thoughts and actions.
2. It can enable you to *focus* the patient's attention on certain aspects of his/her *verbalizations*.
3. It can enable you to *point out* things that the patient finds *difficult to verbalize*.
4. It shows that you are concerned and listening.
5. It lets the sender hear what you heard, so that it can be corrected.
6. By your tone of voice or inflection you can emphasize some aspect of what was said, and you may thereby highlight a hidden meaning in it.

In the following exercise read each patient's statement and write a restatement in the column under *Receiver (dental professional)*. When you have finished, compare your responses with ours.

Sender (patient)	Receiver (dental professional)
Example: I'm very worried about the condition of my son's teeth.	You're very worried about his teeth.
A. I told my wife what you said, and she got kind of upset.	
B. I used to brush my teeth every day, but these last few weeks I have not been able to force myself to do it regularly.	
C. I just wish somebody could tell me something for sure.	

Answer:
A. Your wife got upset when you told her what I said.
   Or: Okay, she got upset.
   Or simply: Your wife got upset.
B. You've had difficulty in brushing your teeth every day.
   Or: You've had difficulty in brushing your teeth lately.
C. You need someone to tell you more specifically what happens to people in your situation.
   Or: You want to know something definite.

CLARIFICATION

Clarification is useful in understanding the patient and in letting the patient know that we really understand what he/she is saying.

In the exercise below, read each patient's statement and write a clarification in the column under *Receiver (dental professional)*. When you have finished, compare your responses with ours.

Sender (patient)	Receiver (dental professional)

Example: When I first came today, they said I would be here for a routine examination or something like that, and I really didn't know what to expect. I've been here by myself for 30 minutes. Having to wait makes me jittery.

When you first came, you thought it would be relatively simple and routine. Being here longer than you expected has caused you to become upset.

A. So then when they told me that this flossing would cure me of my gum problems but when I did it and it hurt and bled all over, I didn't know about it all. I asked my friend and he said he never has any problems with his teeth and he never does anything. That's why I stopped.

B. Doctor, if I let you do the biopsy, I just don't know what will happen then, and I don't like the idea of surgery, either. I mean, what if something happens? I feel worried about you letting some chick give me a shot without telling me. It's all just too much to think about. I mean, I don't know.

Answer: A. You thought from the bleeding and discomfort that the flossing was doing more damage than good.

B. In general, you have a lot of anxiety about the whole procedure.

Interview evaluation

Persons who are concerned with improving and maintaining their interviewing skills will be assisted by systematic feedback and evaluation. This is true for both students and established dental health professionals. Indeed, persons who are concerned with continually improving their communicative skills with their clientele may be "students" of interviewing skills throughout their professional lives.

An interview may be evaluated from several positions. The most important evaluation is from the position of the patient. A practical method of obtaining patient evaluation is for the student to role play an interview with a programmed patient or to have an interview with a real patient. The session should be videotaped. Immediately after the interview the patient and the interviewer view the videotape with a third person, who acts as a facilitator.

When viewing the videotaped interview, the patient and the interviewer will probably recall many thoughts and feelings that were not said during the interview. During any interview there are many thoughts and feelings that are not voiced, because of our minds work much faster than we can verbalize our feelings and thoughts. Therefore, at the beginning of the playback of the videotape, the facilitator should emphasize the ground rules that either the interviewer or the patient may stop the tape any time that anything comes to mind. Once the tape is stopped, the facilitator inquires as to the person's thoughts and feelings at that point. When a thought or feeling is expressed, the facilitator uses nonjudgmental, neutral, probing, understanding expressions like the following to fully understand what took place during the interview:

What were you thinking?

What were you feeling?

What risks were involved in saying that?

What did you want to say?

What had you hoped would happen?

How did you want the other person to see you?

What images did you have then, or what images came to mind?

What did you think the other person was feeling?

Did the other person know how you were feeling?

Were you satisfied with your response? His response?

What got in your way of saying or doing that?

You mentioned earlier that you felt such and such; is that feeling or thought
still with you on the tape?

A second way of evaluating an interview is from the position of the interviewer. Again, the interview must be recorded. When videotape is available, it is preferred. In its absence audiotape is a good second choice.

To facilitate the interviewer's evaluation of an interview, we have developed the worksheet on p. 139. To use the worksheet, the interviewer assigns each of his/her replies a number in the first column. Then, using the criteria at the end of the work sheet, the interviewer analyzes the replies according to type, intent, and success. In the second column the interviewer records the letter that corresponds with the type of the reply. In the third column the interviewer records the number that corresponds with his/her intent in using the reply. What did the interviewer want to happen as a result of the reply? In the fourth column the interviewer rates the success of the reply (by listening to the patient's response to it) on a scale of 1 through 5. If the interviewer gives a low rating to a reply, he/she should place an alternate, improved reply in the fifth column.

Once the student has gone over an interview in this way, he/she may then review the interview with another student or faculty person. Only through this kind of hard work can a person truly develop efficient interviewing skills.

INTERVIEW WORKSHEET *

No. of the reply	Type†	Intent‡	Success§	Alternate, improved reply
1				
2				
3				
4				
5				
6				
7				
8				
9				
10				
11				
12				
13				
14				
15				
16				

*Worksheet may be lengthened as needed.

†*Type*
A. Silence
B. Facilitation
C. Open-ended question
D. Support-reassurance
E. Empathy
F. Confrontation
G. Laundry list
H. Direct question
I. Summary
J. Prescription for action
K. Statement
L. Reflection
M. Problem question
N. Interpretation
O. Bridge
P. Yes-no question

‡*Intent*
1. Focus
2. Facilitate
3. Obtain specific information
4. Change topic
5. Close off topic
6. Clarify what patient means
7. Reassure, support
8. Make a point, teach patient, or state a fact
9. Stop patient's behavior
10. Obtain positive rapport
11. Tell patient what to do
12. Test patient's ability

§*Success*
1. None
2. Partial
3. Acceptable
4. More than hoped for
5. Most possible

139

The third way of evaluating an interview is from the position of an observer. For this type of evaluation we have developed an *interview assessment form.* While observing the interview or the recording of the interview, the observer fills out the form, which is then used for discussion and review with the interviewer. It may also be filed as a record of the progress of the student during a course of study.

The form covers the nonverbal as well as the verbal aspects of the interaction. It focuses on the interview process as well as on the content of the information obtained by the process.

| Date | | | Name of interviewer |

INTERVIEW ASSESSMENT FORM

	Needs improvement	*Acceptable*	*Well done*
Approaches patient			
Greeting, use of name	☐	☐	☐
Seating, physical setting	☐	☐	☐
Degree of control	☐	☐	☐
Purpose of interview	☐	☐	☐

COMMENT:

	Needs improvement	*Acceptable*	*Well done*
Begins biography of problem*			
Facilitates beginning comments	☐	☐	☐
Open-ended questions	☐	☐	☐
Silence	☐	☐	☐

COMMENT:

	Needs improvement	*Acceptable*	*Well done*
Continues chronicle*			
Support	☐	☐	☐
Reassurance	☐	☐	☐
Empathy	☐	☐	☐
Confrontation	☐	☐	☐
Reflection	☐	☐	☐
Silence	☐	☐	☐
Summary	☐	☐	☐
Nonverbal	☐	☐	☐

COMMENT:

*Each item within the section may or may not be used during an interview.

INTERVIEW ASSESSMENT FORM—cont'd

	Needs improvement	Acceptable	Well done
Directs for diagnostic details*			
Direct questions	☐	☐	☐
Laundry lists	☐	☐	☐
Yes-no questions	☐	☐	☐
Suggestive questions	☐	☐	☐
Why questions	☐	☐	☐

COMMENT:

Elucidates each problem			
Location	☐	☐	☐
Quality	☐	☐	☐
Quantity	☐	☐	☐
Chronology	☐	☐	☐
Physical-biologic	☐	☐	☐
Psychosocial	☐	☐	☐
Aggravating and alleviating factors	☐	☐	☐

COMMENT:

Finalizes and closes			
Summary	☐	☐	☐
Closure	☐	☐	☐

COMMENT:

Quality of relationship			
Control	☐	☐	☐
Associates to patient's words	☐	☐	☐
Feelings toward patient	☐	☐	☐
Acceptance	☐	☐	☐
Concern	☐	☐	☐
Interest	☐	☐	☐
Feelings from patient	☐	☐	☐

COMMENT:

Continued.

INTERVIEW ASSESSMENT FORM—cont'd

	Needs improvement	*Acceptable*	*Well done*
Report by interviewer (after interview)			
Verbal observations	☐	☐	☐
Nonverbal observations	☐	☐	☐

COMMENT:

Summary of interview (critique)

_____

Signature of observer

Videotape simulations

The videotape simulation is a most useful technique for helping a student learn about personal communication interactions in professional situations and how to interact in the professional role to which he/she is striving.

This technique combines role playing, videotape, self-confrontation, group support, and group learning. An article by Froelich and Bishop, "One Plus One Equals Three," describes this technique.* The title emphasizes that the outcome in learning is more than what one would expect from just combining role playing and videotape.

A simulation that has been used with dental students is provided in this appendix as an illustration. Members of the class or group are selected to play each role. If persons who are not involved in the class or group are used, the discussion involvement in the simulation is markedly reduced.

The simulation is titled "Abscessed Tooth." The first part of the instructions names the role players and gives the setting of the problem. This information is given to each role player.

The role players meet to make the videotape outside of the class period. They each review the statement of the situation. Then each role player is given his/her special instructions concerning the role he/she is playing. The role players are instructed not to share any information about what is in their special instructions.

After the role players have had 5 minutes to read their instructions, the role play begins. The first scene is of the patient and the dental assistant. The other role players are not allowed to see or hear what is happening during this interaction. The interaction is taped for 2 to 6 minutes—as long as it is productive. The simulation then goes on to the next logical interaction, probably a conversation between the assistant and the dental student. During this interaction the persons playing the patient and the faculty supervisor are not allowed to hear what is going on.

The next scene is between the patient, the dental student, and the assistant. The final scene is between the dental student and the faculty supervisor, either at the patient's chair or in another room, depending on how it would most naturally occur. (The number of scenes, who is in them, and where they occur vary with instructors-directors and what they see happening.)

---

*R. E. Froelich and F. M. Bishop: One plus one equals three, Med. Biol. Illus. **19**(1): 15-18, 1969.

The total time of the videotape is usually 20 to 30 minutes. A simulation of this length provides plenty of material for a 2- to 4-hour class discussion.

It is best to have an interval of at least 24 hours between the taping and the discussion. Such a time interval allows the role players to become less defensive about the role they played and leads to more open discussion and learning. At the beginning of class each student is given a copy of the statement of the situation, and the class discusses the problems that are inherent in the situation for at least 5 minutes before the tape is started. Once the tape has been started, the ground rules are that anyone can stop the tape at any time by saying "stop." The discussion about what has been seen then begins. The learning comes from the discussion, *not* from the tape. If fact, after class, the tape should be erased because it is of little value once the class has gone over it. It will not work with next year's class. They need to make their own tape.

Thus, the session consists of viewing 20 seconds to 2 minutes of tape, discussing it for 10 to 15 minutes, viewing more tape, and so on. It is a fun way to teach, and the discussion is at the level of the particular group's interest and understanding. It works with nonprofessionals and advanced specialists; the only difference is in the level of the discussion that develops.

SIMULATION PROBLEM: Abscessed tooth[*]

Mr. Parker is a 37-year-old wholesale furniture salesman for a local manufacturer. He awoke this morning with a painful jaw and shortly thereafter had draining of pus and blood from the painful area. He needs to be in Springfield this afternoon to set up a display that opens at a meeting tomorrow morning. He is in charge of the setup and the only one who has ever set up this new exhibit. The exhibit has been months in the planning for this important regional trade show. Mr. Parker had taken medicine as a teenager for a heart problem.

Mr. Parker is being seen at 8:30 AM as an emergency referral from the hospital emergency room after having asked the doctor there to pull the painful tooth.

Mr. Stewart is the dental student.

Mr. Anderson is the dental assistant.

Dr. Dunn is the faculty supervisor.

----

[*]Given to all participants and class members.

144

Dr. Dunn*

You pride yourself on being able to manage any patient. All Mr. Stewart really needs is some experience. Show Mr. Stewart how to handle Mr. Parker.

Mr. Parker needs a firm authority figure to set him straight. As you pointed out in a recent lecture, the dentist must be in control of the situation. Mr. Parker should have prophylactic antibiotic therapy before the extraction, and neither you nor the student should be put in the position of being liable for a lawsuit. In your lecture you also pointed out alternatives to treatment, such as referral of the patient, refusal to treat the patient, and so on.

From your experience, reading, and general knowledge, elaborate on the role in any way that you wish. Our purpose is to focus on the issues adherent in the situation.

-----

*Given only to the named role player.

Mr. Anderson*

What is your role? Should you help Mr. Stewart? Should you say something? Do you have any suggestions? After you see what is happening, can you get Mr. Stewart away from the patient and give him some suggestions? How can you help in such a difficult situation?

From your experience, reading, and general knowledge, elaborate on the role in any way that you wish. Our purpose is to focus on the issues adherent in the situation.

-----

*Given only to the named role player.

Mr. Stewart*

Dr. Dunn recently gave you a lecture on the importance of being in control and on the importance of prophylactic antibiotic therapy before the extraction of teeth. In fact, a number of malpractice lawsuits were reviewed in which the dentist had to pay when he did a procedure, at the patient's insistence, that the dentist knew was not wise. Ways of getting control of the situation and alternatives to treatment, such as refusal to treat the patient, referral of the patient, and so on, were suggested.

As you reflect on Mr. Parker, he surely seems pushy, a foot-in-the-door type of salesman who won't take no for an answer.

From your experience, reading, and general knowledge, elaborate on the role in any way that you wish. Our purpose is to focus on the issues adherent in the situation.

-----

*Given only to the named role player.

Mr. Parker*

This regional meeting is very important to you since you expect to get the jump on competitors with a new line of lightweight, easily assembled plastic furniture. This should mean increased sales, production, and personal income. In fact, you hope to double your income from this line of furniture.

You want your tooth pulled so that you can get on the road. You had another tooth like this pulled in Eldon 2 years ago without any trouble and without all of these questions by the student. You are willing to take medication after the tooth is pulled, but you need it pulled to be on your way by 10:00 AM. Don't take no for an answer.

You were hospitalized for 6 weeks at the age of 13 years because of rheumatic fever, edema, and a heart murmur. You took penicillin for 4 years and have not had any trouble since then. You also watch your diet so that you do not spill any sugar in your urine.

Do not volunteer information; be a little difficult; try to cut out all of the student's questions and get him down to the work of pulling the tooth.

From your experience, reading, and general knowledge, elaborate on the role in any way that you wish. Our purpose is to focus on the issues adherent in the situation.

---

*Given only to the named role player.

The following illustrations are the first pages of several other simulations. Make up your own individual specific instructions for these. If you are unable to come up with specific instructions, you may write R. E. Froelich and F. M. Bishop for copies.

SIMULATION PROBLEM: Bleeding gums

Mr. Larson, a 35-year-old store owner, had some bleeding from his gums last summer. Since there is now a dental school in the neighborhood, he has made an appointment for a checkup. Unknown to Mr. Larson, he is "Dr." Munroe's first patient. Mr. Newman, the dental assistant, worked in a private dental office before coming to the dental school. Professor Sharp, a dentist with 25 years of dental office experience, is in charge of the dental clinic and is the supervisor of student work. He was in private practice until 2 months ago, when he quit because of symptoms of angina. Today is Mr. Larson's first visit to the clinic. He was told by the secretary that it "won't take too long." The appointment was for 1:00 PM, and it is now 1:10 PM as Mr. Newman gets Mr. Larson from the waiting room.

SIMULATION PROBLEM: Loose teeth

Mr. Jacobs is a bookkeeper for a local hardware store. He is aware that for some time his teeth have been a "little loose"; that is, he can move them slightly with his fingers. He has shopped around with several dentists who have given him different suggestions; in general, however the suggestions have all involved rather extensive periodontal surgery and expensive splinting (bracing together) of his teeth. It has been suggested that he may loose his teeth within a year or so if he does not have this treatment done. He is reluctant to enter into this extensive treatment.

He is coming for the first time to the dental college to see what the "experts" have to say about his teeth and to see whether there is some way other than surgery and splinting to save his teeth.

Mr. Stewart is a dental student who has been working in the clinic for several months. He understands that the appropriate treatment would be periodontal surgery and splinting. In fact, this topic was covered in a recent lecture by Dr. Dunn.

Dr. Dunn is the supervisor in the clinic this afternoon and will be around to check on Mr. Stewart, as he does with each student in the clinic.

Mr. Anderson is a dental assistant who is in his second semester in the dental hygiene school.

147

SIMULATION PROBLEM: Sore gums

Mr. Laser, a 21-year-old senior college student, has come to the dental office with extremely sore, bleeding gums. He is being treated by Ms. Holmes, the dental hygienist. She has worked for Dr. James for 2 years. Ms. Holmes begins a scaling procedure but then begins to question whether she should be doing this procedure, because of Mr. Laser's discomfort.

Mr. Laser is from out of state and has come to the University to study architecture. He is finding school more difficult than he had anticipated.

Dr. James is a general dentist in this town. He sees many college students as patients. This is his first time to see Mr. Laser. He does not agree with Ms. Holmes' initiative in treating this patient. Usually, he accepts her taking the initiative.

SIMULATION PROBLEM: Rumors in town

Dr. Black has a young but established dental practice in this community of 16,000. Up to this time he has employed an assistant, Ms. Kramer, and a secretary-receptionist, Ms. Casey. Both of these women have been with him for his 6 years of practice.

Dr. Black needed at this time to be relieved of some of the preventive aspects of the practice, so he decided to hire a dental hygienist.

He contacted the state university and hired a young graduate, Ms. Rush, who is attractive, eager to please, and enjoys discussing all aspects of dentistry.

Ms. Kramer is 24 years old and started with Dr. Black as an assistant after high school graduation. Ms. Casey is 43 years old. She is unhappy about the addition of Ms. Rush. A rumor has been going around town about an affair between Dr. Black and Ms. Rush.

Dr. Black is 34 years old. He is married and has two children. He returned to his hometown after 2 years in the navy and has become a prominent person in the community.

A meeting of the office staff has been called for 2 hours from now.

SIMULATION PROBLEM: As the chair turns

Dr. Dennis has been in practice for 15 years in this town of 45,000. Ms. Richards has been his receptionist for 6 years. She acts as office manager, schedules patients, directs patient flow, and orders supplies. Ms. Andrews has been Dr. Dennis' dental assistant for 8 years. She was taught early on the job how to take x-ray films and how to do the basic prophylaxis. Thus, many of the older patients look to her for such care. Ms. Hendricks joined Dr. Dennis' staff 4 months ago as a dental hygienist shortly after she was graduated from dental hygiene school.

Ms. Hendricks has just learned from the patient's record that Ms. Andrews took x-ray films and did the prophylaxis last week on Mr. Myers, a long-time patient. Such treatment by an assistant is contrary to the standard of care Ms. Hendricks was taught in the state dental school.

Ms. Hendricks decides to talk to Ms. Richards about the situation.

Index